# GETTING WELL, STAYING WELL

## EVERYTHING YOU NEED TO KNOW TO GET THE BEST MEDICAL TREATMENT

## GARY GITNICK, M.D, FACG

PROFESSOR OF MEDICINE AND CHIEF, DIVISION OF DIGESTIVE DISEASES
UCLA SCHOOL OF MEDICINE
MEMBER AND PAST PRESIDENT OF THE MEDICAL BOARD OF CALIFORNIA

PHOENIX BOOKS

ISBN-10: 1-59777-539-8
ISBN-13: 978-1-59777-539-7
Library of Congress Cataloging-In-Publication Data Available

Book & Cover Design by: Sonia Fiore

Printed in the United States of America

Phoenix Books, Inc.
9465 Wilshire Boulevard, Suite 840
Beverly Hills, CA 90212

10 9 8 7 6 5 4 3 2 1

# TABLE OF CONTENTS

# PROLOGUE

The healthcare system in the United States is broken. As it continues to deteriorate, obtaining high-quality care is becoming more and more difficult for more and more people. Some can pay exorbitant amounts of money to overcome the increasing obstacles to healthcare delivery, but enrolling in a "concierge medicine" program is a very costly approach that few can afford. Meanwhile, millions of people have little or no access to healthcare, and that is a tragedy.

I wrote this book because I believe that most people can proactively get healthy, stay healthy, and live longer and better, and because I believe that everyone—rich, poor, powerful, weak, regardless of nationality or culture—has the right to excellent healthcare. I am confident that someday a new system will evolve that will provide this universal accessibility. But until that time comes, many people need a guide to help them protect their own interests, advocate on their own behalf, and manipulate the existing dysfunctional system. It is my hope that this book can serve as such a guide and enable people to obtain the high-quality healthcare that they deserve.

# INTRODUCTION
## The Patient-Doctor-Hospital Dilemma

At age forty-seven, Bill had never had a serious illness. Hardworking and hard-driving, he had risen to become a full partner in his large metropolitan law firm. His workload was substantial, his only exercise was an occasional golf game, his vacations were rare, and he seemed to be getting less and less sleep. In the past ten years, he had gained a few pounds each year and had become portly.

Bill's personality had slowly darkened as his workload had increased. He was now less loving, less friendly, less social, and less likeable—and his wife was worried. He was no longer the man she had married. For many months, she urged him to see a doctor, as his only previous medical evaluations had been brief examinations for insurance applications; nothing abnormal had ever been found. After many discussions and arguments, he finally agreed to undergo a physical at my office.

After a detailed history and physical exam, Bill had a series of routine blood tests, a heart stress test reviewed by a cardiologist, a prostate exam by a urologist, and a skin exam by a dermatologist. Despite his obesity, lack of exercise, and diet high in carbohydrates and fat, the only abnormality found was a hemoglobin level bordering on anemia, slightly above the lower limit of normal. As he did not appear malnourished (he was, in fact, overnourished), there was no apparent explanation for his borderline hemoglobin, so additional blood tests were done, and it was found that his serum iron was decidedly low. But when Bill submitted his claim, his insurance company denied payment for the serum iron test, pointing out that there was no indication for it because his other test results had all been within the normal range.

I was concerned as to why a person with no obvious nutritional problem would have a low serum iron level. I advised Bill to have a colonoscopy to rule out polyps or cancer and possibly explain his iron deficiency (as a result of internal bleeding from a polyp or cancer). His insurance company would not preapprove a colonoscopy, pointing out that he was under fifty and stating that there was no real indication for the test. I urged him to have the procedure done anyway. At colonoscopy, he was found to have a lemon-sized tumor on his colon. A biopsy revealed that the tumor was malignant, and he subsequently had surgery to remove it. In spite of an unhealthy lifestyle and a system that denied insurance coverage for the critical tests that eventually saved his life, Bill beat the odds.

Around the same time I met with Bill, I spoke with a friend who had been in good health throughout her fifty-eight years but in the previous year had been diagnosed with breast cancer and had undergone a lumpectomy. Recently, she'd had an abnormal mammogram. Fortunately, a biopsy showed that her abnormal breast tissue was benign. She also had a body-brain PET (positron emission tomography) scan to search for any spreading of the breast cancer, and the scan showed an abnormality in the area of the thymus gland. Her doctor advised her to wait three months and repeat the scan to see whether the abnormality would resolve spontaneously.

When she told me about this, I advised against waiting. I reiterated that the reason to do a PET scan in this situation is to look for malignancy, and that if an abnormality is found, it is imperative to move quickly to prevent the spread of even a small tumor. I suggested that she get a second opinion. She did so and was urged by that doctor to undergo a surgical procedure, at which she was found to have a malignant tumor of the thymus. Fortunately, it had not spread, was well-encapsulated, and was probably completely eliminated by the surgery.

Both of these patients received the wrong advice, and the system failed to provide them with the benefits of good judgment and good practice. We can all see that today's healthcare system does not function properly. Patients, as well as healthcare providers, are victims of its inadequacies and fragmentation, and few patients are sufficiently educated in manipulating the system to protect their own medical interests. Even those who know the right questions to ask may not know where or how to find the answers.

How do you live well, stay well, and live long in good health? How do you find a good doctor? How do you find a good hospital? Do HMOs really serve the needs of their clients? Are PPOs the best alternative? How do you get in to see a doctor expeditiously? How do you know which tests are safe and which are dangerous? When and how do you get a second opinion? How do you protect your own interests? How can you find a doctor who will provide you with the highest quality of care, leave no stone unturned, and make wise decisions, but also communicate clearly, be understanding and thoughtful, provide you with options, and help guide you in your decision-making?

Through patients' stories and several series of questions and answers, this book seeks to confront these issues and provide you with practical information on how to be well, stay well, and get the best care possible out of our existing healthcare system.

# SECTION 1
## Getting Healthy and Staying Healthy

My friend and patient Mike is ninety-two years old, bright, alert, well-oriented, and mentally sharp. He owns and oversees four companies, goes to work every day, and is one of the wealthiest men in our city. He just had his annual physical in my office, and all of his tests yielded normal results: cardiac stress test, carotid duplex scan, and a variety of blood tests. He is trim, at a weight appropriate for his height, has no health complaints, and appears much younger than his actual age.

Mike's father and mother both died in their mid-sixties, and his twin brother also died in his sixties after a life of smoking, excessive drinking, obesity, and depression. I first met Mike in his mid-eighties, when his locker was near mine at the gym. I admired the fact that he usually arrived earlier and departed later than I did, and as we moved from being acquaintances to friends and then to doctor and patient, I grew to admire many more of his lifestyle and health choices.

As a teenager and college student, Mike had not been especially athletic. He did not participate in any group sports or go frequently to a gym. In his twenties and thirties, he worked long hours and acquired several companies that became very profitable, but in his late thirties he felt dissatisfied. He was working so hard that he spent little time with his wife and children. Although he was financially comfortable and had many acquaintances, he had few friends. After one especially difficult weekend in which his business challenges became bitter and his family life was approaching an upheaval, he decided to analyze his situation.

Out of that self-analysis came a determination to change his lifestyle regardless of the cost or effort. He wanted to live long enough to see his children and grandchildren grow up, and he wanted to maintain a loving relationship with his wife. He wanted to look better and feel better. He stopped smoking, refused all alcohol, and started to run each morning. He gradually increased his distance and pace, and he grew to cherish that period of quiet solitude. He found that during exercise, his mind was clearer, and he was able to solve problems and plan ahead without being interrupted.

Mike's weight dropped as his exercise routine increased, and he also adopted a common-sense diet. He avoided carbohydrates and fat and consistently ate healthily, with occasional "treat" rewards. Over a period of eighteen months, he lost more than fifty pounds, ending up within the normal range for his age and height. He found that his business still flourished, and his ability to interact with others was remarkably improved. He felt well, lived well, spent time with his children, and had a "date" with his wife every night.

For the next fifty years, Mike spent at least one hour on aerobic exercise every day. He eventually stopped running because he wanted to avoid the knee and back problems that he saw his friends developing. He switched to using an elliptical machine in the gym, combined with upper body and lower body exercises for muscle strengthening, plus stretching for twenty minutes each morning and evening.

Now, at ninety-two, Mike feels well and is grateful for his good health and functioning, close family life, and successful business. Although he and his brother shared the same genetic background, it is easy to see how one man could die in his sixties and the other could be thriving in his nineties. With that in mind, this section presents some guiding principles in how to get well, feel well, and stay well even as we age.

## WHAT IS SUCCESSFUL AGING?

We are living in a time of unprecedented longevity. Some people seem to become increasingly depressed with age, whereas others are exercising more, traveling more, reading more, and enjoying life more than ever. What makes the difference? I believe a key factor is taking personal responsibility for our health and well-being.

Aging can be time well spent. More people are figuring out how to be as vigorous as possible, maintain their fitness, eat well, manage stress, and minimize age-related disease. Many who used to turn to therapy and plastic surgery are turning instead to meditation and exercise. As a result, more people are enjoying each stage of life and living longer and better than ever in the history of the world. Attention to nutrition, fitness, spirit, and mind is being integrated into wellness programs throughout our nation. Many people today are even finding themselves healthier and happier as they age than when they were young and ostensibly more vigorous.

 WHAT SHOULD I DO TO BE AS HEALTHY AS POSSIBLE AS I AGE?

On the one hand, there are no guarantees. There is no way to promise that you will not get some illness or have an unexpected heart attack or stroke. You can reduce the risk, but you can never reduce it to zero. On the other hand, I do believe that there are three main ingredients to aging healthfully. The first and most important is exercise. The second is nutrition. The third is continually stimulating your mind by reading, thinking, and keeping in touch with the world around you.

##  ISN'T MY HEALTH REALLY UP TO MY GENES? WHY SHOULD I BOTHER TO CHANGE MY LIFESTYLE?

It is estimated that genetic influences account for about 30 percent of the health problems associated with aging—and that lifestyle accounts for 70 percent.

Although we may have genetic predispositions, the risks associated with these predispositions can be reduced by lifestyle changes. For example, if your father, grandfather, and great-grandfather died of heart attacks, you would be wise to control your weight, exercise regularly, monitor your blood pressure, and keep your cholesterol at an acceptable level. If you have a family history of cancer, consider routine screening, as several cancers can be detected early and some can even be prevented from developing beyond a pre-cancerous stage.

Even people with "good genes" can succumb to the health risks associated with obesity, smoking, excess alcohol consumption, poor nutrition, and lack of exercise. Genetic predispositions certainly exist, but in the big picture, your genes account for only a small part of how well or how long you live. The strong influence of environment and lifestyle on health and longevity is undeniable.

**WHAT ILLNESSES ARE DUE TO LIFESTYLE RATHER THAN GENETICS OR BAD LUCK?**

Strokes, heart attacks, several common cancers, many falls and fractures, type II diabetes, hardening of the arteries...the list goes on and on.

 **IF I EAT A LOT, DRINK A LOT, STAY FAT, AND DON'T EXERCISE, SHOULD I ASSUME THAT I WILL DIE YOUNG?**

Not necessarily. Indeed, you may die old, decayed, and decrepit, rather than young and fat. In this era, you can very well live into your eighties and nineties, but your quality of life may be awful unless you pay attention to common-sense health rules. People who are thin and trim, exercise, and eat healthily are more likely to age better and live longer and better.

Our rate of deterioration is determined in large part by how we live. You can age and still function well. It all depends on your focus on healthy living. In particular, you must put daily exercise at the top of your priority list—forget the excuses and just do it.

 **HOW CAN I REDUCE THE STRESS IN MY LIFE? ARE THERE GUIDELINES FOR WELL-BEING?**

There is no magical formula for stress reduction and well-being—I can only give you my own thoughts on the subject. Most of us live stressful lives.

Many of us are self-sacrificing and even feel guilty about attending to personal needs such as relaxation. We often neglect important relationships and postpone gratification. Many doctors believe we would be better off looking more to our own needs.

Accordingly, they recommend the following to patients:

- Exercise. Work toward doing at least one hour of aerobic exercise per day. In addition to this, make time for stretching and relaxation techniques.
- Vacation. Take a four-day weekend every eight weeks and a two-week vacation every six months. You will come back "a new person" and better able to handle your problems.
- Talk and then sleep. Before you go to bed every night, sit down and talk with your spouse or significant other. Twenty to thirty minutes of discussion can work wonders. Follow this by eight to ten hours of sleep—and do not feel guilty about actually getting enough sleep.
- Laugh. Find comedy in life. Be serious when it's important to be serious, but be sure to laugh as often as possible.
- Listen. A good listener is far better than a good talker. A good listener hears not only what is said but also how it is being said and what is really meant.
- Communicate. Make an effort to talk to other people. Strive to be a good communicator. Make eye contact, and when you meet people or when you

leave them, use a handshake or some other form of touch to express your sincerity.

• Meditate. Learn about meditation and use it every day as a self-help tool.

 ## IF DECAYING WITH AGE IS INEVITABLE, WHAT'S THE POINT IN EXERCISING?

Most of our cells are programmed to decay after a certain time, and our bodies are also programmed to replace them. Muscle cells, for instance, are replaced about every four months, blood cells every three months, and bone cells about every two years, whereas platelets are replaced every ten days and taste buds every day. Some organs are even designed to destroy cells while others function to build them.

As part of your immune system, white blood cells called "killer cells" destroy bacteria, cancer cells, viruses, toxins, and other foreign materials in the body. White blood cells also finish off your decaying cells that have been damaged or are undergoing programmed cell death. In addition, white blood cells are involved in the inflammation process that is a precursor to repairing injured tissue. Thus, decay actually stimulates regrowth.

Exercise brings on the inflammation that causes the repair process to move forward. When you exercise, nerve signals are sent out to cause your muscles to contract, and a biochemical signal is sent out to cause your muscle cells to grow. Exercise also facilitates weight loss, better sleep, better blood sugar regulation, and the burning of fat. In turn, you are less likely to have a heart attack, high blood pressure, arthritis, stroke, diabetes, and elevated cholesterol. But if you fail to exercise, decay can take the lead over your body's rebuilding mechanisms.

So, as you can see, there is a natural balance in the body between decay and renewal. To keep these processes balanced in our favor, we should do aerobic exercise every day to stimulate cell death, repair, and growth. Research has shown that the segment of the population that is most fit has one-third the mortality of the population segment that is least fit. When it comes down to living longer versus dying younger, aerobic exercise promotes the former, whereas a sedentary lifestyle promotes the latter.

## IS THERE A SECRET TO LOSING WEIGHT?

Common sense tells us that if fewer calories are going into the body than are being used by the body, the body should lose weight. The simple reality is that weight control must become a lifetime practice. The key is daily aerobic exercise, combined with calorie control, that is best undertaken by eating healthily and cutting portion size. Significantly reducing consumption of carbohydrates such as desserts, breads, and alcohol, avoiding fatty foods such as red meat, and maintaining portion control will inevitably result in weight loss. It happens sooner in some people than in others. Many reach a plateau and need encouragement to be patient, because more weight loss will eventually follow this plateau.

Many doctors believe that people should weigh themselves regularly, and as soon as they see weight gain, take better control of their eating and exercise to return to their previous weight. Many fad diets and weight-loss programs only work while you follow them. People often find that after they stop the diet, or program or "miracle pill," they regain more weight than they lost. Some are even harmful, and none has typically sustained weight loss without an accompanying effort to undertake regular aerobic exercise, calorie reduction, and portion control.

 I DON'T EAT MUCH, AND I PLAY TENNIS AND GOLF REGULARLY, SO WHY CAN'T I SHED MY EXCESS WEIGHT?

Tennis, golf, and baseball are great sports and a lot of fun but are not aerobic—that is, they aren't steady, uninterrupted activities that keep your heart rate up. As soon as you stop moving, the benefit stops. As was mentioned, aerobic exercise is the key. Strength training has its role, but it is aerobic exercise that prolongs your life and is more likely to help you lose weight. Start slowly and set realistic goals—be persistent and have faith. Eventually, as you build up your aerobic exercise regimen, you will feel better, lose weight, and look better.

 ## HOW MUCH AND WHAT KIND OF EXERCISE SHOULD I DO TO KEEP MYSELF IN GOOD SHAPE FOR LIFE?

Work up to doing at least one hour of aerobic exercise, seven days a week. Aerobic exercise is exercise in which you are constantly in motion and maintaining an elevated heart rate: examples include swimming, walking, jogging, running, or riding a stationary bicycle, regular bicycle, or elliptical machine. You may build up to this over a period of time, but eventually, aerobic exercise must become a daily ritual that you commit to for life.

In addition, you want to keep your muscles and bones strong. With professional guidance, you may wish to undertake regular strength training with weights or machines. Stretching is also very helpful. Learn stretches from a professional and do them in the morning and at night. The aerobic exercise, however, is the most important—the others are "icing on the cake."

Find out what your weight should be for your age and height, and make that your goal. If you exercise in the described ways, and at the same time reduce the amount of calories you consume, it will be easier to lose your excess weight and keep it off. If you diet without exercising, however, the odds are against you.

I'M OLD, OVERWEIGHT, AND OUT OF SHAPE. I LOVE TO EAT AND DRINK, AND I HAVEN'T REALLY EXERCISED SINCE HIGH SCHOOL. SHOULD I TAKE ANY PRECAUTIONS BEFORE I START AN EXERCISE PROGRAM?

See your doctor before you start an exercise program, as you need to know whether you have any condition that would make it unsafe. Then, when you first start to exercise, get into it slowly. Give yourself a long-term goal and increase the intensity and length of your exercise over time. Be sure to discuss your exercise regimen with your doctor at your subsequent annual physicals.

 I SMOKE, I'M OVERWEIGHT, I HAVE HIGH BLOOD PRESSURE, I EAT TOO MUCH SALT, I DON'T EXERCISE.... SHOULD I CHANGE ALL OF MY BAD HABITS AT ONCE OR TACKLE ONE AT A TIME?

A recent study addressed this issue in a large number of patients. Remarkably, those who were asked to change all of their bad habits at once, rather than one at a time, tended to do better.

 HOW SHOULD I CHANGE MY EATING HABITS FOR BETTER HEALTH AND FITNESS?

Use common sense and eat foods that you know are good for you. Avoid fast foods, foods that contain lots of fats, and most simple carbohydrates such as sugary and overprocessed foods (including products made with white flour). Aside from the occasional glass of red or white wine, which may be good for your heart, avoid drinking alcohol, as it is loaded with calories and burdens your liver.

Also, reduce the volume of food you eat. When you eat out, a helpful strategy is to convince your significant other to share meals with you. You can split an entrée and still enjoy good food while keeping your volume under control.

## WHAT FOODS ARE ESPECIALLY HEALTHY?

Recent data suggests that "Mediterranean foods" such as figs, salmon, beans and other legumes, nuts (especially almonds and walnuts), and whole-grain bread are especially good for us. In general, it is recommended that we eat lots of fruits and vegetables. Green, leafy vegetables, for instance, are thought to lower some cardiovascular risks. Spinach, endive, and romaine, as well as other foods high in folate or folic acid, are thought to help reduce or slow the cognitive problems associated with age. The omega-3 fats in seafood are reported to lower the risk of heart disease and many other conditions. Whenever you can choose fish over red meat, choose fish. Olive oil is another healthful fat. Increasing data also suggests an advantage of eating whole grains rather than overprocessed bread, pasta, rice dishes, and cereals—remember that oats and other whole grains are rich in fiber.

 **IF I PREFER NOT TO DRINK ALCOHOL, HOW CAN I STILL GET THE CARDIOVAS-CULAR BENEFIT OF RED WINE?**

An alcoholic drink is not really necessary, because grape juice is just as good at lowering your cholesterol levels. A recent study has shown that compounds in grape juice can also stimulate a chemical process called nitrous oxide reduction, which aids in keeping blood vessels elastic.

 **SHOULD I HAVE AN ANNUAL PHYSICAL?**

Many doctors believe that men and women should see their family doctor at least once a year. The kinds of tests needed at that time vary from person to person according to the patient's age, family history, and any symptoms or existing conditions. It is a good idea for your doctor to get to know you by seeing you regularly. It is also wise to be screened for specific illnesses depending on your particular risk factors.

 **WHAT'S THE BEST WAY TO FIGHT EVERYDAY GERMS?**

Sneezing, nose-wiping, coughing people touch doorknobs, handrails, books, and everything else, and there's no getting away from these germs.

Wash your hands. Studies show that people who regularly wash their hands get fewer gastrointestinal and respiratory illnesses. Hand-washing is probably the most important thing you can do to protect yourself from bacterial infections such as those caused by staphylococcus (staph), as well as many other infectious diseases.

 ## WHAT ARE THE TRAITS OF PEOPLE WHO LIVE TO BE 100 OR MORE?

About 40,000 Americans are 100 years old or older. Eighty-five percent of these people are women, only a few of these people are overweight, and most do not smoke. Eating right and staying active, challenging the mind, and exercising devotedly seem to help. The New England Centenarian study and a similar Japanese study show that genes are also predictors of who will live to 100 and who will not. Some centenarians, for instance, have a particular gene that lowers the risk of autoimmune and inflammatory diseases.

There are, of course, dramatic exceptions to the "rules," such as a French woman named Jeanne Calment who smoked until she was 117 and habitually ate chocolates until her death at 122. Nevertheless, with or without "good genes," a healthy lifestyle seems to make a big difference.

**IF EXERCISE AND EATING RIGHT ARE SO IMPORTANT, WHY DID A GOOD FRIEND OF MINE, WHO WAS IN EXCELLENT CONDITION, EXERCISED DAILY, AND ALWAYS ATE HEALTHY FOODS, DIE UNEXPECTEDLY IN HIS LATE FIFTIES?**

Although many diseases can be prevented, many occur unpredictably. There are no guarantees that doing everything right will ensure a healthy, long life, but it greatly improves your chances. It has been estimated that about 30 percent of illnesses develop in spite of all that we try, but that about 70 percent can be prevented by healthy living. A regimen of daily aerobic exercise, strength training, healthy diet, and weight control improves your chances of having good health and a long and good life.

# SECTION 2
## Choosing Your Doctor and Managing Your Managed Care

Although a high income is certainly helpful, access to excellent healthcare is becoming increasingly limited for people at all income levels. Largely because of rapidly decreasing reimbursements from managed care providers and insurance companies, doctors spend less time with each patient in order to see more patients and thereby generate more income. It is hard to reach these overloaded doctors by phone or schedule an appointment, and the limited time available in appointments may lead them to make mistakes or overlook things.

As the healthcare system becomes dominated by what is called cost-effective medicine, it moves toward providing more patients with less service—and care becomes progressively more difficult for any patient to obtain. In response to this situation, some doctors have elected to practice what is called concierge medicine. This section discusses how to be your own healthcare advocate, make reasonable healthcare decisions, and increase your likelihood of getting great healthcare.

## SHOULD I USE AN HMO, A PPO, OR SOME OTHER FORM OF HEALTH INSURANCE?

HMOs (health maintenance organizations) charge a set annual or monthly fee for coverage of medical services. Their incentive is to provide care, but at the same time, ensure profitability by spending as little as possible on drugs, tests, procedures, and consultations. Thus, the HMO physician is charged with providing care that minimizes costs to the HMO—in some instances, creating an obvious dilemma for the physician, who is also ethically charged with providing good care to the patient.

HMOs are often very good when you are healthy—that is, they provide vaccinations, regular check-ups, and appropriate testing at appropriate intervals. In some instances, HMOs (or their patients) get into trouble when less expensive procedures, tests, or drugs are utilized that are often, but not always, equivalent to their more expensive counterparts. HMOs vary in quality when you are sick or have a complex or costly illness.

A good test of any HMO you may be considering is to ask some subscribers whether that HMO worked well for them at a time when they were very sick. Alternatively, you may be acquainted with a physician who can give you some insight into the quality of various HMOs. Many states have a Web site (sometimes sponsored by the Department of Health Services or the State Board of Managed Care) that provides an assessment of HMO quality based on objective criteria.

The problem is that what may be good for most people may not be good for all people. The concept of cost containment as practiced by HMOs is not inherently bad—unless the cost-based decisions delay or prevent effective and expeditious care. Some HMOs are good, some are bad. It is a case of "buyer beware." In most instances, HMOs only approve care given by the doctors they employ. Each HMO contract specifies particular criteria or circumstances under which the HMO will pay for the use of "outside" physicians or emergency rooms.

PPOs (preferred provider organizations) give patients more choice. PPOs usually promote the use of a list of physicians who have signed a contract to reduce their charges to a required level in exchange for having patients referred to them by the PPO. In most PPO contracts, the patient also has the option of seeing physicians not on the PPO's list, but the portion of the professional fee covered by the PPO may be significantly reduced, or payment may be denied altogether.

You may wish to purchase another form of medical insurance or use the Medicare system to have more choices of physicians and facilities, but this is sometimes more costly than utilizing an HMO or PPO cost-containment program.

## 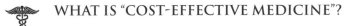 WHAT IS "COST-EFFECTIVE MEDICINE"?

Cost-effective medicine weighs the likely benefit of a consultation, procedure, test, treatment, or drug against the costs of these elements in a large population of patients. HMOs, PPOs, medical groups, federal or state governments, and insurance companies may arbitrarily determine a cut-off level above which they consider that the cost is not justified by the benefit. This may result in restricting the use of expensive treatments, encouraging the use of less costly treatments, and denying requested services if it is determined that the "cost-effectiveness" or "cost/benefit ratio" does not justify their use.

## WHAT IS "CONCIERGE MEDICINE"?

In a concierge medicine program, each patient is charged a fee, usually annually—for example, $25,000—in return for a number of special arrangements pertaining to healthcare services. Concierge fees can range from $2,500 to $100,000 per year above the amount that the doctor would bill to an insurance company for medical care. In addition to the concierge fee, patients pay out of pocket or through insurance for the costs of the doctor's time and services, specialists' consultations, tests, and treatment.

In return for this financial investment, the doctor guarantees convenient, around-the-clock care by attentive staff. Most doctors who practice concierge medicine limit their number of patients to ensure adequate time and attention for each patient's evaluation and treatment. Many also reserve time slots during the day to handle unplanned appointments. In most instances, the doctor's patient coordinator can schedule an appointment quickly and conveniently around the patient's schedule.

Other guarantees include that the patient will be expeditiously referred for appointments with consultants and will be met by the doctor at the ER, in case of emergency. The concierge doctor is accessible around the clock, on weekends, and on holidays. In addition to making regular services easily available, concierge medicine often provides patients with added services such as an escort by a care coordinator to the doctor's office and to wherever tests are to be performed.

In some concierge practices, blood tests and electrocardiograms are conducted in the doctor's suite, rather than requiring that patients go to a lab or other offices. Following any evaluation, the doctor calls the patient to discuss the test results and also sends the patient a booklet that documents these results and provides general healthcare information relative to any abnormalities or conditions found.

If hospitalization is necessary, a patient care coordinator will often assist with arranging the admission, escorting the patient, and obtaining a room. The concierge doctor or a colleague will oversee the patient's care in the hospital.

## IF I'M LOOKING INTO A CONCIERGE MEDICINE PROGRAM, WHAT QUESTIONS SHOULD I ASK THE DOCTOR?

Here are some questions that may help in your selection process:

- Do you limit your practice? If so, for how many patients do you care, and how many patients do you usually have in the hospital?
- What are your credentials?
- Do you work with specialists who also provide your patients with easy access to care? If so, in what fields do these specialists practice?
- Which hospital has given you admitting privileges?
- Can you provide references from existing patients?
- Are you participating in continuing medical education programs?
- Do you attend national meetings and educational courses?
- Can I count on you to be my advocate if problems arise in the hospital or during outpatient care?
- Will your staff make appointments for me when you recommend that I have tests or see other doctors?
- Will your staff advocate on my behalf to expedite appointments?
- Will your staff arrange my appointments and tests in such a way that I spend as little time as possible away from my regular activities?
- Can I determine how many tests I want to have on a given day?

## HOW DO I FIND A GOOD PRIMARY CARE DOCTOR?

It has become a real challenge to find a primary care doctor who provides all the services that most people want. Very often, the economics of medical practice require doctors to limit the time spent with each patient in order to ensure enough patient volume to cover overhead costs and yield a profit. Furthermore, with the expansion of multispecialty clinics and medical groups, many doctors and patients overfocus on subspecialty care, so patients often go to a subspecialist for everything from headache to stomachache. These patients, however, may not have one doctor who is in charge of their care, serves as their advocate, and helps interpret the recommendations of other doctors.

Unfortunately, many primary care doctors are overworked. To handle their crowded waiting rooms and large patient volume, they may delegate a large portion of patient care to "physician extenders" such as nurse practitioners or physician assistants. Accordingly, it is not unusual for many patients to receive most of their healthcare from a physician extender rather than a doctor.

Nevertheless, there are still many good and even great doctors out there who truly are dedicated and provide excellent care. Look for a primary care doctor who is not only intelligent, experienced, calm, patient, and compassionate, but also has connections with the best specialists in your area. Primary care doctors have usually specialized in family medicine or internal medicine after training in general medicine.

Medical subspecialists such as cardiologists, gastroenterologists, hematologists, and others sometimes provide primary care as well. Subspecialists are first trained to be internists and then undertake subspecialty training.

The best way to identify the most competent doctors is to ask any doctors of your acquaintance for the name of their primary care or family doctor or internist. If you find that difficult or impossible to do, then ask other healthcare professionals to recommend a doctor. Nurses can be especially knowledgeable as to who is good, who is bad, who is responsive, and who has a good bedside manner.

Asking friends is not a very reliable way to assess the competence of a primary care doctor, as most nonmedical people judge doctors simply on personal appearance and whether they are nice. Nevertheless, you do want someone with whom you can have good "chemistry" and communication. So when you've identified a doctor who is seen as competent by his or her colleagues, it is then worthwhile to ask friends, relatives, and other patients about that doctor's personality, responsiveness, and accessibility, and whether the office is efficient.

Once you find a potential candidate, check the Web site of your state's medical board for anything recorded about that doctor (start at the board's home page and follow the links to the information of interest). Adverse comments reported by a state medical board are generally reliable. Few boards, however, are allowed to disclose all complaints or settlements, and the absence of adverse comments may not ensure that your doctor is competent. Many state medical boards are required by law to list only the most serious or costly malpractice or disciplinary actions, and many do not disclose actions that were dropped or settled. Therefore, it's relatively easy for a doctor to pass this board "sniff test"—but if he or she does not, it's likely that the mistakes made were serious and multiple.

Thus, with the recommendations of other doctors, feedback from other people, and information from the medical board Web site, you can generally determine the quality of your potential doctor. Other factors that may be helpful include whether the doctor is board-certified and/or affiliated with a school of medicine. Full-time faculty members usually have good credentials and maintain a high degree of familiarity with current medical literature. Of course, medical school faculty can be as good, bad, nice, or not nice as any other doctor in private practice.

## HOW DO I FIND A GOOD PHYSICAL THERAPIST?

Most orthopedic surgeons can refer you to a physical therapist with a proven track record. Another route is to ask your doctor or other doctors you know for the name of any physical therapist whom they utilize. Generally, a doctor will pick the best for his or her family. Remember that a physical therapist needs to provide treatment under the direction of a physician, and it is usually best to have your physician write a prescription for the specific kind of physical therapy recommended for your needs.

## SHOULD I AVOID GETTING MEDICAL CARE FROM DOCTORS WHO ARE CLOSE FRIENDS OR RELATIVES?

Generally, yes. The closer a doctor is to you, the less objective he or she may become. It can be difficult to evaluate relatives' or dear friends' complaints with objectivity, especially when we are concerned about their well-being. It is quite human to block out the more serious or unusual possibilities. Accordingly, it is best to see doctors who are friendly but distant enough to maintain objectivity.

## IF I'M TOLD I NEED TESTS, WHAT QUESTIONS SHOULD I ASK BEFORE I AGREE TO HAVE THEM DONE?

Ask questions such as the following, and persist until you get satisfactory and understandable answers:

- What does this test measure?
- Why do I need this test?
- What could happen if I do not agree to have this test?
- Are there alternatives to this test that are just as good and/or have fewer side effects?

 IF I'M TOLD I NEED SURGERY, WHAT QUESTIONS SHOULD I ASK BEFORE I AGREE TO HAVE IT DONE?

The following list of questions may be useful in discussing a proposed surgery with your doctor:

- Why do I need this surgery?
- What alternatives are there to having the surgery?
- Is there a significant difference in outcomes between the alternative treatment and the surgery?
- What data is there that indicates surgery is the best treatment choice?
- What would happen to me if I refuse this surgery?
- What are the risks involved with this kind of surgery? How likely are they?
- If there is more than one possible approach to this surgery (such as minimally invasive laparoscopic surgery rather than a standard open operation), which approach is thought to produce the best outcomes, and which approach do you advocate for my particular case?

## WHEN SHOULD I ASK FOR A SECOND OPINION, AND HOW DO I GO ABOUT GETTING ONE?

In my family, we ask for a second opinion whenever a serious diagnosis is proposed, a controversial treatment is recommended, a treatment plan does not seem to be working, symptoms persist or worsen, or surgery is recommended. Ask your physician to invite another physician who is an expert in the field to offer a second opinion. A good doctor will not be insulted by a request for a second opinion. After all, if the second opinion concurs with the first doctor's, that simply makes him or her look better, and if the second opinion does not concur, unnecessary errors may be avoided.

A second opinion should be obtained from a physician who is not in practice with the doctor who offered the first opinion, so it will not be influenced by any financial relationship or partnership. When you are an inpatient, the second opinion will need to be given by a physician who has what is called "privileges" at that hospital or who is granted temporary permission to evaluate you there. When you are an outpatient, it is often wise to ask your physician to arrange for a second opinion from a physician affiliated with a different medical center to ensure objectivity. Above all, in both circumstances, the second opinion should come from a physician with experience in the problem being evaluated.

## DO DOCTORS REALLY CARE ABOUT THEIR PATIENTS? SHOULD I CARE ABOUT MY DOCTOR?

Most patients do not realize how the progress of their illness and their response (or lack of response) to treatment affects their physicians. Doctors frequently think about and worry about their patients. After all, we went into medicine because of our desire to help patients, and because we found dealing with aches, pains, and illnesses to be more interesting and more challenging than almost anything else. Most doctors really do care—though few patients realize that they actually do have an impact on their doctors.

 ## WHEN IT COMES TO HEALTHCARE ACCESS, DOES THE SQUEAKY WHEEL GET THE GREASE?

Not necessarily. It is important to remember that although it may be necessary for you to advocate in a firm but friendly manner for your own healthcare, that is not equivalent to being verbally abusive or rude. Good doctors know when patients are too sick to be polite, and they will handle this in a professional manner—but some patients have their mind set on abusing the doctor or other medical personnel. Patients perceived as rude and unfriendly may find that doctors will spend even less time with them and may order more tests and consultations to protect themselves from any possible problem or litigation.

MY DOCTOR TALKS TOO FAST, USES WORDS THAT I DON'T UNDERSTAND, AND GIVES SUCH VAGUE INSTRUCTIONS THAT WHEN I LEAVE THE OFFICE, I DON'T KNOW WHAT I'M SUPPOSED TO DO. WHAT SHOULD I DO ABOUT THIS?

To better understand your diagnosis and treatment plan, ask your doctor to show you diagrams and write down your diagnosis as well as written instructions for you to take home. If there is still a problem, call your doctor after you've had your appointment to request a clearer explanation.

 I NEED A LOT OF TESTS, SO WHY IS MY DOCTOR URGING ME TO HAVE THEM ALL DONE AS AN OUTPATIENT RATHER THAN PUTTING ME IN THE HOSPITAL?

If you are ambulatory—that is, able to get around, even if you require assistance—it is wise to avoid unnecessary hospital stays. A hospital can be a dangerous place. Hospital-acquired infections, errors in giving drugs or other treatments can occur in spite of the staff's diligent efforts to prevent them. If you can avoid hospitalization by opting for outpatient care, do so. If you must go into the hospital for testing, get in and get out as quickly as you can.

 HOW DO I GET HEALTHCARE FOR A WORKER IN MY HOUSEHOLD WHO IS SICK AND UNINSURED?

For the immediate problem, if your employee does not qualify for Medicaid and is a member of the "working poor," your options are limited. In a true emergency, any ER is obligated to provide care, even if that care is not reimbursed. County healthcare facilities are usually obligated to provide even non-urgent care. They often bill the uninsured patient and refer unpaid accounts to collection agencies, but care is usually provided. Waits may be long, quality may be variable, and communication may be limited in such situations.

For future needs, either pay for your employee's health insurance yourself or insist that he or she obtain it. It may be worth your while simply to pay a local physician to provide healthcare until your employee gets health insurance.

 WHAT IS A LIVING WILL, AND HOW DOES IT DIFFER FROM HEALTHCARE POWER OF ATTORNEY AND A DNR ORDER?

When you cannot speak for yourself, a living will gives instructions to your healthcare team regarding your wishes for your care. Laws regarding living wills vary from state to state. Technically, you can write your own living will, but practically speaking, it is often a good idea to have an attorney do it. You'll have to make some difficult decisions as to under what circumstances you do or do not wish to be resuscitated and under what circumstances you do or do not wish to have invasive procedures or life-extending machinery.

Be sure to give copies of the document to each of your doctors and at least two of your relatives.

In granting healthcare power of attorney, you appoint a specific person to make medical decisions for you when circumstances prevent you from doing so. If you have a living will, this person is charged with ensuring that its directions are followed, but in situations that the living will may not adequately cover or when no living will exists, this person is designated to make those decisions if you are unable to. This frees other people from needing to join in the decision-making about your care and often prevents unnecessary conflicts in a stressful time. It is wise to discuss these issues with your family, so you can make your desires clear and prevent unnecessary consternation. For married couples, the spouse is usually designated as having healthcare power of attorney. It is a good idea to talk about this with your spouse and your physician, as they both need to be comfortable with your decision and their roles. Laws regarding healthcare power of attorney vary from state to state, and your doctor or hospital can probably provide you with the necessary state-specific forms. Some states require the signature of a witness.

If you do not have a living will and have not designated a person to hold your healthcare power of attorney, you still can indicate your wishes when being admitted to a hospital. If you request a DNR ("Do Not

Resuscitate") order, no efforts will be made to preserve your life if your heart stops or if you stop breathing. If you do not request a DNR order, resuscitation will be attempted.

When developing these various doctrines, try to be as specific as you can. Do you wish to be connected to a ventilator that will pump air in and out of your lungs? If you are unable to eat, do you wish to be fed intravenously or through a tube in your stomach? If your heart stops or if you stop breathing, do you wish CPR (cardiopulmonary resuscitation) to be attempted? Keep in mind that as long as you are able to communicate, you can reverse any of your prior instructions.

If you wish to be an organ donor, you need to document this as well. Sign an organ donor card, which is available at most hospitals and most doctors' offices, and verbally notify your doctors, relatives, and friends of your desire to donate your organs. Some states allow you to sign your consent to be an organ donor on the back of your driver's license.

 ## HOW DO I UNDERSTAND MY MEDICAL BILL?

Medical billing and collections are typically a mess. For an outpatient appointment, your physician's billing company bills you directly. The charge for your physician's professional services is based on his or her determination that the consultation was average, complex, or extended. Outpatient laboratory tests are usually billed separately, with the bill sent directly by the lab or the radiology or nuclear medicine office. For some imaging tests, you are charged a basic fee for the test as well as a professional fee for the radiologist's interpretation of the result. Many doctors and laboratories utilize a fee structure established by the Medicare Administration, even for services to patients who are not receiving Medicare.

Hospital bills are often very difficult to understand. The bill shows a separate charge for every service, every medication, and every hospital day. However, you may also receive a separate bill for the professional fee of every physician involved in your evaluation and care, from your main doctor to the radiologist, pathologist, or any other consultant. Some medical centers conquer the problem of multiple bills by combining the charges for all of their services, including fees for hospital-based physicians, in a "super bill."

Regardless of the quality of a medical center or physician's office, billing mistakes are often made. A wise patient will call the billing office for an explanation of any unclear charge.

WHY IS THERE A DIFFERENCE BETWEEN THE CHARGES TO INSURANCE COMPANIES AND CHARGES TO UNINSURED PATIENTS?

Physicians and hospitals establish a fee for each procedure and service. Those who accept Medicare usually must use a fee structure approved by the Medicare Administration. Most medical insurance companies negotiate significant reductions in fees for procedures or services provided by a hospital or healthcare professional. These negotiated contracts enable patients insured by that company to utilize that hospital or doctor based on those fee reductions. Uninsured patients, however, are often charged full fees without any insurance-negotiated discounts.

 HOW DO I KEEP AN ORGANIZED MEDICAL RECORD SO I HAVE INFORMATION AVAILABLE FOR A DOCTOR OR EMERGENCY TREATMENT?

The AARP (American Association of Retired Persons) has a medical record template that helps you organize and store your health history and medical records. It is online at www.aarp.org.

 CAN I HAVE COPIES OF MY MEDICAL RECORDS? HOW DO I GO ABOUT GETTING THEM?

You can and you should. Your medical records are your property. Your doctor's office files on you, as well as your hospital records, actually belong to you. You may not understand all of the language used in these records, but it is a good idea to keep a copy in a master file at home in case the information is ever needed on short notice. If you have been hospitalized, it is wise to request—in writing—a copy of your medical records from that hospitalization. Similarly, when you have tests as an outpatient or see any consultants, ask for copies of the test results and the consultant's report to keep in your master file.

The law is clear on the point that medical records are the property of the patient. Nevertheless, for the physician, hospital, or lab, sending out medical records to patients who request them is a tedious, time-consuming process, and records may not be made available as quickly as they are needed. If there is a problematic delay, you must be your own advocate or ask your doctor to advocate on your behalf.

In most instances, you need to sign a release of information form, which authorizes and instructs the holder of the records to provide them to you or to a physician or medical facility. A follow-up phone call to the medical records department may expedite getting your records sent. If not, ask to speak to the department supervisor and request his or her help. Go as high in the system as necessary for assistance. If anyone says that you are not entitled to your records, firmly notify the person that the law clearly establishes the records as your property (many low-level staff members may not know this).

If you participate in a concierge medicine program, you should need only to sign a release of information form when you first enroll; thereafter, your doctor's staff should be able to obtain any required records expeditiously. In addition, the staff should provide you with a copy of your medical records held in their office.

 ### IF I'M TOLD MY MEDICAL RECORDS WERE LOST OR AREN'T AVAILABLE, WHAT SHOULD I DO?

It can be quite frightening to find yourself in an emergency, or hospitalized, and unable to obtain your prior medical records. If your doctor has died or retired, the doctor who took over the practice will often retain copies of your records. When hospitals or other facilities such as outpatient radiology units, chemistry labs, or imaging units are uncooperative in finding and providing your records, go as high as you can in that facility's medical records department, requesting—if necessary, demanding—that copies of your records be provided expeditiously, after you have signed a written release. Persistence pays off. You may need to make some phone calls, but those records are your property. If necessary, an attorney can advocate on your behalf.

## IF I FIND AN ERROR IN MY MEDICAL RECORDS, WHAT SHOULD I DO?

Bring the error to the attention of your physician. If he or she agrees that the statement or other information in the record is incorrect, contact the healthcare professional who made the erroneous entry, and request—in writing, if necessary—that the record be amended and that the amended record be included in your file.

## WHAT IS HIPAA?

In April 2003, Congress passed HIPAA, the Health Information Portability and Accountability Act. This law guarantees your right to review your medical records, request changes to your records if inaccuracies are found, and keep copies of your records. HIPAA also protects your privacy by preventing keepers of your records from disclosing any elements to anyone without your written consent.

If your privacy is violated, you can file a complaint with the responsible party or the Department of Health Services Office for Civil Rights: call 800-368-1019, or go to www.HHS.gov/ocr/hipaa. Although you have the right to request that disclosure of your medical records be restricted, existing laws may prevent your doctor or hospital from honoring that request in certain circumstances. For example, doctors are required to report all instances of certain communicable diseases to the Department of Health.

In appraising the information on a Web site, < at the three letters after the dot in the site's ress. A "com" site is usually a commercial entity, therefore it may or may not be reliable. An "edu" is affiliated with an educational institution, and refore the information provided is probably urate, although it may not always be up-to-date or ensive. A Web address ending in "gov" is a vernment site and usually a reliable source. address ending in "org" represents a nonprofit ity and often, but not always, provides reliable ormation.

Reliable Web sites indicate the source of the ormation, identify the material's authors and their alifications, and provide references to accompany edical facts and figures. Another important criterion recency. If the site has not been updated in a long ne, the content is not likely to be current. Also, if the e contains advertising, question whether it is onsored by a pharmaceutical company and perhaps cordingly biased.

 **WHEN I AM TOLD THAT A CLINICAL TRIAL OR OTHER MEDICAL STUDY SHOWED SUCH-AND-SUCH, HOW DO I KNOW WHAT IS RELIABLE AND WHAT TO BELIEVE?**

When assessing the credibility and value of a edical research report, some detective work is

HIPAA can also, unfort
you by preventing your doctor
information with other doctors o
without your prior written cor
would be wise to give your doct(
ahead of time, to share your ir
doctors involved in your care.

 ### IS THE INTERNET TH
### MEDICAL AND HEALT
### FOR THE LAYPERSON

No and yes. The Inter
publication of unproven concepts
have not been subjected to "pe
recommendations without substa
them and without review by ex
critical of the data or methods. On
Internet does enable you to acces
well-supported information. The I
issue is to judge your source.
established by a major medical
medical school, or sponsored by a
organization, or reflects informat
medical textbooks, it is generally (
other hand, the information is b
individuals or business entities, be
to remember that online health ir
completely wrong, outdated, unned
or slanted to sell a product.

involved. In medical school, doctors learn to analyze studies, assess the strengths and weaknesses of research reports, and judge what to accept and what to question. This can be very difficult for the layperson. However, here are some pointers:

- Determine whether the study was performed at a reliable institution.
- Determine who paid for the study and whether precautions were taken to ensure that the investigator's assessments would be independent and unbiased by any commercial or other sponsors.
- Determine whether the study was large enough to yield meaningful data. It is better to draw conclusions from data obtained from a large number of people who were selected for the study, utilizing clear-cut criteria and including an appropriate control group, rather than to rely on data obtained from only a few people.
- Determine whether the participants were put in the treatment and control groups randomly so no prejudgments affected group assignment and influenced the outcome.
- Determine whether the control group was followed prospectively along with the treatment group and whether the groups were comparable before the study began; at the very least, they should have been similar in regard to race, age, gender, and disease stage.

- Determine whether the study was "double-blind"— that is, if possible, that the participants did not know whether they were receiving a treatment or a placebo, and that the investigator also did not know which participant received which until after the study.
- Determine whether side effects were found in one or both groups, what the side effects were, and what their frequency was.
- Determine whether the differences found between the groups were described as "statistically significant"—that is, different enough not to have occurred by chance, so appropriate and meaningful conclusions can be drawn from a statistical standpoint.
- Determine whether the study's follow-up period was long enough to demonstrate a truly reliable long-term outcome and evaluate any potential long-term complications.

Finally, it is probably wise not to put too much stock in the results of a study until another study performed by other investigators has confirmed those results.

# SECTION 3
## Surviving Outpatient Care

Arturo grew up in an unstable and impoverished home in East Los Angeles, surrounded by violence, gangs, and the drug culture. A high school teacher urged Arturo to work with a mentor from the Fulfillment Fund, which provides young people with college access programs and a variety of social services. He and his mentor, Sam, eventually developed a close personal relationship.

Arturo had always been in good health, but at age seventeen he experienced headaches with increasing severity for two months. At the local free clinic, he spent two hours in the waiting room before being seen (for less than ten minutes) by a medical resident, who examined him and told him to take a non-aspirin pain reliever. But the headaches persisted, and when Arturo eventually told his mentor, Sam arranged an appointment with his own family's internist.

After a three-week wait, Arturo and Sam went to the doctor's office at 10:00 a.m. as instructed. The waiting room was packed, but the doctor had not yet returned from his hospital rounds. At 11:30 a.m., they were called to an examining room. About twenty minutes later, the doctor entered, took a brief history, and performed a brief physical exam but did not perform any neurological assessments. He assured them that he could find no obvious physical problem but would order blood tests. Arturo and Sam waited at the downstairs laboratory for another thirty minutes before Arturo's blood was drawn.

The test results were not available until ten days later. When Sam called the doctor's office, a nurse told him that all of the results were normal. Meanwhile, Arturo's headaches worsened, and Sam decided to take Arturo to a neurologist at his own expense. There was a four-week wait for an available appointment.

After a two-hour wait at the office, Arturo was evaluated by a neurologist, who told Arturo and Sam that there were clear-cut neurological signs of a problem and several tests were necessary. A CT (computerized tomography) head scan appointment was not available for a week, and the results were not available for another week after that. When Sam called for the results, the neurologist refused to discuss them on the phone and insisted that Arturo come for a return appointment.

Ten days later, Arturo and Sam arrived for the appointment and waited for an hour and a half. The neurologist then told them that there was a large tumor made up of blood vessels and involving a major portion of the brain. He said that in his opinion, it was inoperable and fatal, but that he could arrange for Arturo to see a neurosurgeon who might have better ideas. Three weeks later, the neurosurgeon told Arturo and Sam that the tumor was inoperable because of its extent and location and nothing could be done. After discussing this with friends, Sam decided to get another opinion. Two weeks later, Arturo was seen by a second neurosurgeon and again told that the situation was hopeless.

A doctor happened to sit next to Sam at a Fulfillment Fund committee meeting, and he told the doctor of the horrible situation confronting this young man who had turned his life around, only to be diagnosed with an inoperable, fatal brain tumor. The doctor invited them to his office the next day, where one of the staff escorted them to their academic healthcare center to see a prominent neurosurgeon specializing in vascular tumors. The neurosurgeon did a thorough exam, reviewed the CT scan, and ordered a variety of tests. He then told Arturo and Sam about an experimental procedure that had resulted in remarkable improvement in some patients.

Sam convinced Arturo and his parents to have the procedure done. The surgeon donated his services and Sam paid the hospital costs. The surgery took eight hours. Within a month, Arturo was symptom-free and had no neurological deficits. Since then, he has completed college and entered graduate school, the tumor has not recurred, and he has remained in excellent health.

Let's compare Arturo's experience with a life-threatening condition to Jim's experience with a routine physical. At age sixty-five, Jim is a successful media mogul who works most hours of most days, travels by private jet, and lives in a West Los Angeles estate. For fourteen years, he and his family have participated in a concierge medicine program. For an annual fee, in addition to the costs of tests and professional fees, they have direct "24/7" access to their doctor and his staff. Jim knows that the doctor usually takes his calls immediately, unless the doctor is involved in an emergency, and then he almost always calls back within minutes. He occasionally calls with specific health complaints and is seen expeditiously, usually on the same day. Every few weeks, the doctor calls to see how he is doing.

Jim had canceled his annual physical on short notice twice in four weeks, but then his schedule finally allowed him to allocate two half-days for the examination. Convenient parking was arranged, and he was met at the entrance to the doctor's office building by one of the patient coordinators. Had this been his first visit, the doctor would have performed a complete medical history and complete physical exam before any testing. However, because of their years of association and periodic phone contact, they could expedite the evaluation and associated blood tests. After his exam and tests, the doctor called Jim and explained the results, and the doctor's office sent him a booklet also describing the nature and results of the tests.

For many people less fortunate than Jim, outpatient healthcare in the United States has virtually become a matter of survival of the fittest. Without his mentor's persistence as his advocate, Arturo might not have survived. The difficulty in obtaining appointments, the long waits, and the hasty evaluations all reflect a broken healthcare system that failed him for more than four agonizing months. This section discusses obstacles in outpatient care and provides advice on what to anticipate and how to confront the problems that often arise—forewarned is forearmed.

 ## WHO HAS THE POWER TO MAKE THINGS HAPPEN IN THE DOCTOR'S OFFICE?

The doctor is often the most powerful person in the office. In a medical group, the doctor who is the managing partner has great authority. At the staff level, the office manager usually directs all other employees. The scheduler is very important in determining whether you are seen quickly or in the distant future. The back office nurse is usually closely associated with both the doctor and the patients and has an important role in facilitating doctor-patient interactions. A receptionist may interact with patients as they wait but does not strongly influence the other activities of most medical offices.

## HOW DO I GET THE COOPERATION OF MY DOCTOR'S STAFF?

First, be nice. A confrontational approach may have adverse consequences. Many employers, including doctors, have a policy of supporting their staff unless multiple complaints occur or consequences are egregious. If you need to be firm, do so in a friendly manner and do not be condescending. An occasional gift to the staff (such as candy, flowers, or a basket of cookies or muffins) will be remembered in the future.

## HOW DO I GET AN APPOINTMENT SOONER RATHER THAN LATER IN A BUSY DOCTOR'S SCHEDULE?

Appointments with doctors often are made on a first-come-first-served basis. However, most doctors expedite appointments for patients who have more serious health complaints. If you feel that your complaint falls into this category, but the doctor's staff refuses to alter the schedule, request that the doctor call you to assess the urgency of your evaluation. Alternatively, a letter or email to the doctor will often do the trick. Whatever you do, be nice to the staff. The scheduler is simply doing his or her job at the direction of the doctor, and making an enemy will only result in more problems. If you do get an earlier appointment, a small gift sent to the scheduler in appreciation could go a long way the next time.

If you need to see a specialist or subspecialist, your primary care doctor will be more effective than you will in obtaining an appointment. Ask your doctor, or his or her staff, to request the appointment on your behalf and to emphasize the importance of a time sooner rather than later.

Many concierge medicine practices utilize a network of consulting specialists who agree to adjust their schedules for the benefit of concierge patients. If you participate in a concierge program, your doctor's staff should handle the details in getting you convenient appointments with consultants.

 HOW OFTEN SHOULD I GET A PHYSICAL EXAM, AND WHAT TESTS SHOULD I GET REGULARLY?

Although many doctors believe that annual physicals are not cost-effective, I think it's a good idea to be evaluated by your doctor once a year even if you aren't experiencing any symptoms. Doctors have differing opinions as to which tests should be done annually. Some feel that all patients who have a family history of serious illnesses—for example, ulcerative colitis, Crohn's disease, or malignancies such as breast or colon cancer—should be screened regularly for those conditions. Doctors also disagree on how often adults should have cardiac stress tests, screening blood tests, or colonoscopies.

Many doctors like to see patients every year. With younger patients, the appointment may not entail much more than discussion and a physical exam, unless there is a prior history of a serious illness in the patient or in the family. Some doctors usually recommend that patients over forty years old have: full annual physicals including a complete history and exam, a mammogram for women, a cardiac stress test, a head-to-toe skin exam by a dermatologist, a prostate exam by a urologist for men, and a number of screening blood tests, as well as periodic colonoscopies.

 WHEN I HAVE A SYMPTOM THAT WORRIES OR FRIGHTENS ME, SHOULD I GO TO MY FAMILY DOCTOR OR DIRECTLY TO A SPECIALIST?

It is usually a good idea to keep your family doctor in the loop. However, the cost of care from an internist versus a subspecialist is not very different. Accordingly, a phone call to your family doctor to express your concern about a symptom and discuss a referral to a specialist is often wise.

## WHAT MAKES A "GOOD" PATIENT

"Good" patients prepare ahead of time for doctor's appointments, making it easier for the doctor to understand their problem, find the cause, and plan a treatment. They think through each of their health complaints and symptoms as well as their personal and family medical histories. They disclose all medications, remedies, and supplements they are taking. They bring copies of test results and other relevant documents.

Good patients respect the doctor's time. In answering questions, they try to be complete and accurate but also concise. They ask questions at the end of the history and physical exam, not during the course of the process. They realize that the squeaky wheel does not necessarily get the grease. They respect an educated opinion—however, that does not mean that they do not seek a second opinion.

Perhaps most importantly, good patients comply with the medical advice given and the treatment recommended—not blindly, but having obtained enough information to make sound decisions about their healthcare. (Unfortunately, many patients do not take their prescribed medications or do not adhere to the dosage and timing instructions, which can lead to serious problems.)

## HOW SHOULD I PREPARE FOR MY VISIT TO THE DOCTOR?

If this is your first visit, the doctor will need to take a complete history and do a complete physical exam. Thinking about your visit in advance and writing out the relevant information described below will enable the doctor to better understand you and your health complaints—and will also save a lot of valuable time that could then be used to answer all your questions. And even if this is not your first visit, preparation will facilitate your communication with your doctor and ensure that your appointment is time well-spent on your healthcare.

List all ongoing and new symptoms, and be prepared to discuss them. Record when you first noticed them and any ways they've changed since their onset. Prepare the list chronologically to show how your symptoms evolved. Think about ways to describe them so the doctor can really understand how you feel.

Itemize your medical history of previous illnesses and surgical procedures, including their dates (or approximate dates). List all medications you are taking and the doses of each. Be sure to include any herbal or alternative medicines on that list, as well as vitamin, mineral, or food supplements. Record any allergies, especially to any drugs, and be sure to notify your doctor.

For your family's medical history, provide your grandparents' and parents' significant illnesses and their ages now or at the time of their death. List any significant illnesses in your children and other members of your family.

Obtain copies of your medical records as well as test results, x-rays, or other imaging studies you may have had, and bring these to your appointment. And don't forget to bring a list of your questions (see below).

 ### WHAT QUESTIONS SHOULD I ASK WHEN I GO IN FOR A DOCTOR'S APPOINTMENT?

Think about your concerns, make a list, and bring the list to the appointment. It is better to ask questions at the end of your meeting, after the doctor has reviewed your history and performed a physical exam. Although tests may still be needed to reach a firm diagnosis, you can ask your doctor what conditions he or she is considering and how serious those might be. You can also ask about the tests being performed or planned and any risks that might be associated with them.

Once your doctor provides a firm diagnosis, ask about the natural course of your illness. What can you expect in the future? What signs or symptoms should trigger a call to the doctor? Do you need to be concerned about passing the condition to others? How can you help yourself recover? Ask about any medications your doctor is prescribing for you, what their side effects may be, and whether they will interact with any drugs you're currently taking.

Finally, ask your doctor whether you can call or email about any additional questions you or your family may have after you've gone home and thought about your discussion.

 ## HOW DO I AVOID A LONG WAIT IN THE DOCTOR'S WAITING ROOM?

Some degree of waiting is generally inevitable (unless you are in a concierge medicine program). One approach is to call the doctor's office a few hours before your scheduled appointment to ask how long a wait you can anticipate and whether the doctor is behind in his or her schedule for that day. Depending on what you find out, ask whether you can adjust your appointment time so that you'll have little or no wait.

Another strategy is to talk to anyone you know who sees this doctor, and find out about his or her waiting room practices. Some doctors, for example, have a slew of patients arrive at 10:00 a.m. and wait to be seen one at a time, and then do the same thing again starting at 1:00 p.m. Others schedule two or three patients in the same time slot to avoid having any unfilled time due to cancellations or no-shows. In either scenario, the first patient to arrive is likely to be the first patient seen by the doctor. If you don't relish the prospect of arriving at dawn or skipping lunch, send an email to the doctor explaining your time constraints, and ask if it would be possible for him or her to evaluate you at a convenient time but with a minimal wait.

Most doctors schedule people sequentially into specific time slots—but we all know that some patients take more than the allotted time and cause a build-up of delay as the day goes on. In this case, perhaps the best you can do is call ahead so you know what to expect, and then bring a book or magazine along.

If you participate in a concierge medicine program, appointments are typically established specifically to avoid waiting. You'll usually be able to arrive at the scheduled time, give your name, and then promptly enter the doctor's office and begin your meeting. Occasionally, of course, an emergency may cause a delay.

 ## HOW DO I GET MY DOCTOR TO SPEND MORE TIME WITH ME?

Good doctors are usually busy. Therefore, doctors often must limit the amount of time they spend with each patient, especially in a managed care situation. However, this limited time is not always sufficient for the patient's care, comfort, and questions.

Call, email, or write to your doctor and ask whether your upcoming appointment can be scheduled in a manner that will allow some additional time for you to get your questions answered. Be friendly and get your doctor to like you. Avoid confrontation and try to be understanding of his or her schedule and needs. If possible, ask to be the first patient in the morning or the afternoon, as the first patient is likely to have more time with the doctor before the schedule starts to bog down. After your appointment, send the doctor a thank-you note or even a small gift. Such gestures of appreciation will be remembered.

If you participate in a concierge medicine program, your doctor's schedule should be designed to enable him or her to spend adequate time with you. Most concierge doctors limit the number of patients in their care and the number of appointments in a day to ensure enough time to meet with each scheduled patient.

 ## WHAT SHOULD I DO AFTER I LEAVE THE DOCTOR'S OFFICE?

If your doctor recommended tests or advised you to see a specialist or other healthcare professional, make—and keep—those appointments. If your doctor does not call you with the test results within the specified time period, call his or her office and ask for the results. If any questions arise, your symptoms worsen, or you think you're having side effects from medications, call your doctor and actively seek a prompt response.

 ### HOW DO I AVOID LONG WAITS WHEN I HAVE TO GO FOR TESTS?

As with doctor's appointments, it is often wise to call ahead to ask how long a wait to expect. Depending on the answer, you can also ask whether there is a better time for you to come for your test. If the staff offers no help or hope, bring a book or magazine along to pass any waiting time.

If you participate in a concierge medicine program, your doctor or his or her staff may have already interceded for you to avoid a long wait, but check with them to be sure, and remind them if necessary. A concierge doctor often provides a staff member to escort you to testing offices or facilities and ensure that your tests are done expeditiously.

 ### HOW ELSE CAN I SAVE TIME IN OUTPATIENT TESTING?

You can try to arrange the appointments to take your tests sequentially on a single day, thus avoiding multiple visits to the laboratory or imaging center and also enabling you to take less time off from work. Some tests, however, cannot be done on the same day as others. For example, scans that require intravenous or orally administered dye may interfere with one another.

If you participate in a concierge medicine program, your agreement should include expeditious and convenient scheduling of tests to save you time.

 HOW DO I GET REPORTS OF MY TEST RESULTS QUICKLY?

Unfortunately, this may be difficult. Although results for most blood tests, x-rays, and scans could realistically be available in a day or less, some laboratories are slow in reporting the results of even routine tests. To speed the process, your doctor might have to call the lab rather than wait for the report to be mailed or faxed to the office. Ask your doctor if he or she can call you about your results as soon as they are available. However, some doctors will only provide test results to patients on a subsequent face-to-face visit rather than by phone.

If you participate in a concierge medicine program, a usual part of the agreement is the expeditious reporting of test results as they become available.

 WHAT SHOULD I DO IF MY DOCTOR DOESN'T CALL ME BACK?

In a medical emergency, of course, call 911. Otherwise, call the doctor's answering service, and ask for the doctor to be paged directly to the service until the doctor calls in (if the doctor is paged to your number, the service has no way of knowing whether the doctor responded). It may also be worthwhile to send an email to your doctor, who may see it while using a computer or pick it up on a cell phone. If your doctor is regularly unresponsive, you need to find another doctor.

If you participate in a concierge medicine program, an essential part of the agreement is that your doctor will take your calls except when seeing another patient, unless you indicate that your call is urgent, in which case you should have immediate access. In most instances, if the doctor cannot take your call right away, he or she should call you back within minutes or certainly on the same day.

 IF I'VE BEEN GETTING MOST OF MY HEALTHCARE FROM MY GYNECOLOGIST, AT WHAT POINT SHOULD I MOVE MY GENERAL CARE TO AN INTERNIST OR FAMILY PHYSICIAN?

The sooner the better. Gynecologists should provide gynecological services. Internists and family practitioners are trained to manage general medicine and handle numerous conditions ranging from sore throats and urinary tract infections to serious illnesses such as cancer. It is my opinion that everyone, regardless of age, should have a family doctor or internist to provide regular physicals and to turn to when symptoms develop.

Let me share a cautionary tale to illustrate my point. A woman in her early thirties was free of any symptoms when she saw her gynecologist, who found no abnormalities. Subsequently, she had an annual physical with an internist, who examined her neck as a routine procedure and felt nodules on her thyroid gland, which turned out to be malignant. This simple examination saved her life. Even without any apparent symptoms, her cancer was caught early enough to be cured, and it has not recurred.

 WHEN I VISIT MY DOCTOR, HE ASKS WHAT HE CAN DO FOR ME. I RESPOND, HE MAY BRIEFLY EXAMINE THE PART OF MY ANATOMY IN QUESTION, AND THEN HE USUALLY RAPIDLY WRITES OUT A PRESCRIPTION. SHOULDN'T DOCTORS REALLY TALK TO PATIENTS?

Yes. A doctor should methodically review each complaint you are presenting, the history of each symptom, your medical history, and the type and dose of any medication you are taking. He or she should also ask a series of questions reviewing all of your body's systems. Then, after performing an appropriate physical exam, the doctor should: give you his or her impression and possible diagnoses, recommend any tests needed to establish the diagnosis, and describe the most appropriate treatment and its associated risks and benefits.

The best medicine usually comes when doctors have time. However, in a broken healthcare system, with the pressures of seeing large volumes of patients to obtain adequate reimbursement and meet the goals set by the administration of the clinic, group practice, or HMO, this kind of thorough assessment often falls by the wayside. If you can find a doctor who takes the time to conduct a complete history and physical exam, ask appropriate questions, and discuss tests and treatments, you are very fortunate. This is a doctor to cherish.

 ## IS IT NECESSARY TO TREAT EVERY SYMPTOM AND CONDITION?

No. Many symptoms and conditions are neither life-threatening nor significant, and unneeded treatment exposes the patient to undue expense and possible side effects. It is not necessary to treat every ache, pain, sniffle, or cramp. However, it is necessary to treat such conditions as high blood pressure and diseases of the kidneys, liver, heart, and lungs. Your doctor can advise you as to when medication is truly needed or when you might be better off putting up with a temporary symptom or two.

**IF A PROBLEM THAT STARTED OUT SEEMING MINOR GETS WORSE, WHEN SHOULD I CALL MY DOCTOR?**

The sooner the better. Patients often do not realize their risks until they speak with their doctor. Doctors can be much more helpful in preventing the progression of an illness or other problem if they get involved early in its course, as treatments are more effective the earlier they are given.

Here's a cautionary scenario: "About a week ago, I think I got a spider bite on my right forearm. Over the next few days, I scratched it and it blew up to become red and elevated. Yesterday, a red streak started moving up my arm toward the inside of my elbow. Should I call my doctor?" The doctor's response: "Your bite is probably infected from scratching. The red streak probably indicates infection spreading up your arm, and there is a potential risk of the infection getting into your bloodstream. You should have called me when you first noticed the bite, and certainly when it became red and swollen, and you'd better call now."

 **IS THERE ANYTHING WRONG WITH ASKING A DOCTOR'S ADVICE AT A SOCIAL EVENT?**

Yes. To give you good advice, a doctor should know the history of your health problem, take the time to ask questions, and examine you. In fact, most states require by law that a doctor perform a history and physical exam before prescribing a treatment. Furthermore, federal law prohibits any doctor from discussing your healthcare issues within earshot of other people. (Exceptions to that, of course, are discussions within earshot of other healthcare personnel involved in the exam or treatment and within earshot of family/spouse/advocates authorized by the patient to hear it.)

A doctor also has the right to private time and a break from work-related topics during social events. As nice as a doctor may be when trapped in an impromptu consultation, it is likely that he or she would prefer not to discuss medical issues outside of the office.

 ## IS IT WRONG TO CALL MY DOCTOR AT HOME IF I HAVE A MEDICAL ISSUE?

Yes—unless you've been specifically instructed to by the doctor or his or her staff. Doctors (and their families) are entitled to private time. Getting away from work and having time to relax is as healthy and necessary for doctors as it is for anyone else. Invading a doctor's home life with phone calls is rude and inappropriate.

On-call systems are set up to manage patients' medical issues outside of their doctors' working hours. If the problem is minor, the covering doctor can easily help you, or your doctor can get back to you during his or her next workday. If the problem is major, the covering doctor can handle it by phone or in person in the ER.

**I'VE BEEN USING SEVERAL PHARMACIES FOR MY MEDICATIONS BECAUSE OF CONVENIENCE AND COMPARATIVE COSTS. IS THAT A PROBLEM?**

If you get medications from several pharmacies without each pharmacy knowing about the other drugs you are taking, you deprive yourself of a very important benefit: being warned about possible drug-drug interactions. For instance, taking two particular drugs together may be harmful, or one drug may lessen the effectiveness of the other. There may also be interactions between herbal medicines or between drugs and herbal medicines taken together. A pharmacist from whom you obtain all of your medications will be able to spot such potential interactions and can help you determine what the relative risk may be.

 **WHAT SHOULD I DO WHEN A HOME HEALTH NURSE IS SUPPOSED TO VISIT, BUT THEN I DON'T GET A CALL, SHE DOESN'T ARRIVE, AND CALLING THE NUMBER I WAS GIVEN LEADS TO A MACHINE THAT DIRECTS ME TO ANOTHER NUMBER THAT DOESN'T ANSWER?**

Home health services are usually contracted out by hospitals or sometimes owned by medical centers. Weekend and holiday scheduling is especially difficult and errors are easily made. Very often, the issues are not with the nurses but rather with their supervisors or the administrators above the supervisors. When you call with a problem, go as high in the system as necessary to get the care to which you are entitled, and do not give up. If you can't get through to the home health company, call information or check the Internet for any alternate phone numbers. If the home health service was directed to you by a medical center or other institution, call that institution's page operator or after-hours number, and talk to the on-call administrator.

When a doctor's wife needed a specially timed infusion, the home health nurse was excellent, but it turned out that his wife's name had not been put on the weekend schedule by the administrative office. He called the medical center and asked the page operator to connect him with the supervisor in charge of home health. He finally reached that supervisor after several calls, and she did not have his wife's name on the schedule either, but she was able to correct the situation.

 I KNOW MY BROTHER IS AN ALCOHOLIC, AND I THINK HE MAY BE A DRUG ADDICT, BUT HE DENIES IT ALL. HOW DO I DO AN INTERVENTION?

You cannot do it yourself. First, contact a professional addiction specialist, who may be able to design an intervention or may refer you to an interventionist. The specialist or interventionist will encourage you to gather those people closest to the person you are concerned about, including friends and relatives. With the help of this professional intermediary, that group can confront the alcohol- or drug-addicted person and stand some chance of convincing him or her to enter a rehabilitation program. It is unlikely that you will be able to accomplish this without the help of a professional. Your physician should be able to refer you to an addiction specialist who can guide you through this very difficult, painful, but important, intervention process.

# SECTION 4
## The Emergency Experience

Michael was a seventy-four-year-old retired attorney with a complicated medical history. He was diabetic and had recently started using insulin. Ten years previously, a large benign pancreatic tumor had necessitated surgery to remove most of his pancreas and a portion of his intestine, with reconnection of the bile and pancreatic ducts to the small intestine. Two years later, a large abdominal hernia (a protrusion of intestine through the prior surgical incision) was surgically corrected. Six years later, he developed abdominal pain and vomiting and was found to have a bowel obstruction due to adhesions (scar tissue surrounding the bowel), which again required surgical correction.

Two years later, Michael awoke one night with nausea, vomiting, and pain around his belly-button. His abdomen became distended and he vomited every ten to fifteen minutes. He and his wife decided to wait it out, assuming that he had food poisoning, and he continued to vomit several times an hour until dawn.

By 9:00 a.m., his vomiting was less severe and less frequent, but he still had abdominal distention and pain. He called his physician, who was not available, and the physician assistant recommended that he go to the emergency room.

As a member of a PPO (preferred provider organization) that separated its outpatient and in-hospital physicians, Michael knew that he would not see his family practitioner at the ER or hospital. When he arrived in the ER, the reception area was packed, the waiting area had standing room only, and gurneys carrying seriously ill patients were lined up in the hallways of the treatment area. Ambulance attendants, police, and patients' relatives and friends filled any available space.

Michael still had abdominal pain, distention, and intermittent vomiting but waited patiently in line to give his name, address, telephone number, and complaint to the receptionist. He waited in another line to see the triage nurse, who eventually interviewed him as to the nature, duration, and severity of his condition and took his pulse, blood pressure, and temperature. He was then directed to the ER business office, where he waited in yet another long line to receive a series of lengthy forms in tiny print and have the clerk make a copy of his insurance card.

Having already been at the ER for over an hour, Michael was sent back to the waiting area, which was still standing room only. An hour later he asked the receptionist when he might be seen, and she didn't know but said that many people had been waiting for over six hours. An hour later, he called his physician's office again and explained his situation to a physician assistant, who advised him to stay in the ER. He asked the physician assistant to talk to the ER doctor, but she declined, saying that was not her role. Every hour thereafter, he asked the receptionist when he'd be seen and received the same non-answers.

Finally, Michael and his wife left the ER, drove directly to the airport, got on a commuter flight to Los Angeles, and called a well-known doctor's office from the airport. One of the patient coordinators pulled up a summary of Michael's prior admission to their hospital for the bowel obstruction due to adhesions. She reached the doctor by cell phone and cross-connected him to Michael, who was en route in a rental car being driven by his wife. The doctor told him to meet him at the hospital's ER.

The doctor called the surgeon, who had operated two years before, to request that he come down to the ER to evaluate Michael after the initial exam. Next he called the ER director, who said it was a "zoo" but then agreed to reserve an ER bed when the doctor explained the patient's history and likely bowel obstruction for which treatment had now been delayed more than ten hours. The doctor also notified the ER radiologist of the probable need for x-rays and alerted the triage nurse that Michael would need to be brought quickly to the reserved exam room.

The doctor met with Michael when he arrived. Following a brief history and a thorough physical exam by the ER resident and then by the doctor, he was wheeled to radiology for abdominal x-rays and then brought back to see the surgeon. The surgeon, ER resident, ER director, and the doctor reviewed the case and agreed on the presence of a partial bowel obstruction. They decided to pass a nasogastric tube (through the nose down to the stomach) to try to decompress the abdomen by suction. Michael would be monitored and given intravenous antibiotics, so if his condition didn't improve within six hours, or if any changes indicated the need for urgent surgery, they were prepared to operate.

No bed was available in the intensive care unit, so they obtained a private room and called in a private duty nurse. The nasogastric tube was connected to a wall-mounted suction apparatus to begin the decompression treatment. Meanwhile, the blood test results were rapidly obtained, and it was clear that Michael was severely dehydrated and needed intravenous fluids. Within six hours, his abdomen was much flatter, his vomiting stopped, and he was far more comfortable. His blood sugar was brought under control, and the next day he was discharged.

In this case, Michael was first the victim of an overloaded, inefficient, unhelpful emergency system and subsequently the beneficiary of a busy but much more user-friendly system. What if something like this happens to you? This section will help prepare you to advocate on your own behalf in an emergency situation and to enlist others to advocate for you as well.

 ## WHAT CAN I DO NOW TO PREPARE FOR AN EMERGENCY LATER?

- If you have a drug allergy or a serious illness such as coronary artery disease or diabetes, wear a Medic Alert bracelet or necklace so ER doctors can get instant information about you if you are unable to communicate.
- Next to your telephone, keep the phone numbers of the local poison control center, your physician, the nearest ER, and someone who you would want to drive you to a doctor or hospital in the event of illness or emergency.
- If there are children at home, teach them to dial 911 in an emergency.
- List all of your medications and their doses.
- List all of your current diagnosed illnesses and treatment.
- List all of your past illnesses and operations, including approximate dates.

- List all drugs to which you are allergic as well as drugs with which you've had side effects, and list the side effects.
- Keep all of your medications in their original containers, and keep those containers in a plastic bag to be easily taken with you in an emergency.
- Write down the directions to the nearest ER.

 ### HOW DO I DETERMINE WHICH EMER-GENCY ROOM IS BEST?

Often you must simply go to, or be taken to, the nearest ER. You can, however, judge ERs in your neighborhood or city by various criteria. The better facilities have a variety of backup physicians who are usually in the hospital. You want an ER that can handle emergency neurosurgery and vascular surgery such as emergency angioplasty for blocked arteries. If you are experiencing symptoms of a possible stroke, you want an ER that can provide emergency thrombolysis to dissolve clots that may be blocking blood vessels to the brain.

In general, you are better off at an ER classified as a trauma center, as these are especially capable in handling injuries from auto accidents, falls, gunshot wounds, or other accidents. An ER classified as "level three" is most qualified to handle serious problems. Level three ERs also usually have easy access to cardiologists, gastroenterologists, and other subspecialists in the hospital. Information about an

ER's qualifications can usually be obtained on the Internet by visiting www.qualitycheck.org.

 HOW SHOULD I HANDLE AN EMERGENCY?

In a true emergency, the first thing to do is call 911. If you feel that the problem does not require ambulance transportation or is not truly life-threatening, then you can be driven to an ER. At the first available opportunity, call your doctor (or ask a friend or family member to call) to report the situation and where you are going. Ask the doctor to call the ER's director with information about your medical history and to remain in touch with the treating doctor as your management progresses.

If you participate in a concierge medicine program, your doctor will probably meet you at the ER and facilitate care provided by the ER staff.

 WHAT INFORMATION SHOULD I BRING WITH ME TO THE EMERGENCY ROOM?

You will need your insurance card, and it would be very helpful to bring the above-mentioned lists of your current conditions, prior illnesses, drugs, and allergies. You may not have the presence of mind to gather all of this together in the stress of the moment, but do the best you can. It helps to prepare ahead of time, just in case. If you plan ahead, you can also make sure that a family member or friend knows where you keep this information and can bring it to the ER for you.

## HOW SHOULD I TRAVEL TO THE EMERGENCY ROOM?

Call 911 and have paramedics take you in an ambulance, or have a friend or relative drive you if you feel that your problem is not that urgent. People who drive themselves to an ER often do not make it.

 ## HOW SHOULD I HANDLE A CROWDED EMERGENCY ROOM?

Be nice, friendly, and firm. Hysteria and confrontation usually make things worse. Ask the triage nurse or the person at the receiving desk how long the wait is likely to be. If the estimated wait is not acceptable, ask the nurse to make sure the ER doctor is aware of the seriousness of your condition. Above all, call your own doctor and ask him or her to talk to the ER physician to expedite your care.

If you participate in a concierge medicine program, your doctor will probably meet you at the ER and facilitate your care.

 ## WHO'S WHO IN THE EMERGENCY ROOM, AND WHAT WILL THEY DO FOR ME?

The personnel in most ERs work as a team. Each staff member has a predetermined function, and most are well-trained and efficient. Usually, the first person you will meet is a receptionist who will record your name, address, telephone number, and complaint and then refer you to a triage nurse. The triage nurse will ask you more detailed questions about the nature of your complaint and decide, based on its seriousness and severity, whether you should be seen immediately or after other patients.

Depending on that outcome, at some point you will be referred to the ER's business office, where a clerk will make a copy of your insurance card and ask you to complete a form providing additional basic information. Eventually, you will be called into an examining room where a nurse will take your pulse, blood pressure, and temperature, listen again to your complaint, and then post your name, complaint, and room number on the ER board.

If you are at a teaching hospital, a medical student and an ER fellow may see you next. These doctors in training will take a history, perform a physical exam, and report their findings to an attending physician. (There is often an advantage to having multiple people take your history, as even an inexperienced doctor may pick up a clue that others have missed.) Eventually, the attending physician will also take a history, perform a physical exam, and order blood tests, x-rays, scans, or whatever is appropriate. He or she may be overseen by an ER director, whose job is to ensure that the ER functions efficiently and that the most serious problems are handled first.

## WHAT ARE MY RIGHTS AS A PATIENT VISITING AN EMERGENCY ROOM?

For information on the rights of ER patients, see www.emtla.com.

d abdomen. He was then wheeled to a waiting
here he remained for an hour until another
took him back to his room.

A few hours later, a young doctor came in and
e was taking over the next shift. Unfortunately,
outpatient records still could not be found, and
octor needed more information. For the next
minutes, more questions were asked and
ered, and another perfunctory chest and
men exam was followed by a promise to "get to
ottom of this." About thirty minutes later, a floor
e came in to start an intravenous line and stuck
r in five different places with no success, so he
he'd get somebody else to start the IV, but it
ht take some time as they were very short-handed.

Dinner never came. After two hours, a nurse
rted the IV. Peter's family visited until visiting hours
ded. He read a book for a while but was distracted
the noise from the hallway. The nurse came back to
ke his vital signs and then left, leaving the door
en. He tried to sleep, but the noise and his fears
bout his health kept him awake, and nurses came in
very four hours to take his vital signs.

A CT scan was performed the next day, but
when he asked for the results, the technician said he
had not looked at the test. Two days later, Peter asked
again and was told the CT scan was normal. He then
underwent an upper GI (gastrointestinal) series for

# SECTION 5
## The Challenges of Hospitalization

Peter is a fifty-eight-year-old restaurant
manager whose mild diabetes is controlled by low-
dose insulin. He had been obese all his life until fifteen
years ago, when he underwent a stomach-stapling
operation and subsequently lost 125 pounds. His
health dramatically improved, as his high cholesterol,
blood sugar, and blood pressure normalized, and his
previously constant fatigue was replaced by more
energy than he'd had in years. However, when eating
meat or raw vegetables, he could easily overfill his now
small stomach and develop vomiting. He found that
overeating also produced symptoms including
heartburn, a bitter taste, and the reflux of stomach
contents. Accordingly, he was usually careful about
what he ate.

When Peter developed occasional difficulty
swallowing and regurgitation shortly after swallowing,
he called his doctor, but the first available
appointment was four weeks later. As his swallowing
difficulty became more frequent and the regurgitation

more severe, he became dehydrated and eventually could tolerate only liquids. He was finally evaluated at a large multispecialty clinic by a doctor with whom he had previously had brief and generally unsatisfactory meetings. The doctor was distant and formal and under pressure to see his daily patient quota.

In the fifteen minutes allotted for a return patient visit, the doctor listened to Peter's complaint, asked a few pointed questions, and performed a brief abdominal evaluation. Peter needed to be hospitalized to improve his nutrition and find the cause of his swallowing and regurgitation problem. Unfortunately, the hospital was full and six ER patients were already waiting overnight to be admitted, so Peter's admission was delayed by two days.

When Peter arrived at the hospital, the admissions area was packed. He stood in line for fifteen minutes, spoke with the receptionist, and took a seat in the waiting area. Over an hour passed before he was called into an admissions cubicle to sign documents and provide his insurance card, even though the card had already been presented and the same information recorded in a hospital referral document when his admission was arranged two days before.

It was another thirty-five minutes until an orderly wheeled him to his hospital room, where an unsmiling nurse instructed him to put on a hospital

gown and await her r
came in and took hi
temperature. When P
nurse, he was told tha
working elsewhere in th
assistant left, no one cam

Finally, a woman
and said she would be his
hospital, as the doctor he'c
assigned to the hospital ro
to a "glitch," Peter's medic
transferred, and the com
information about his recen
unfortunately, the doctor ex
more new admissions, plus oth
needed to be brief. She sper
asking about his symptoms and
doing a physical exam. When Pe
conclusions, she said she had to
and then left.

It was now lunchtime, but it
Peter to eat the food on his tray wit
Two hours later, a nurse came in a
red, one white, and two blue pills.
about these medications, she said ;
find out what they were for. A few m
orderly came to wheel Peter to x-ray, w
for forty-five minutes until x-rays wer

chest a
area, w
orderly

said h
Peter'
the d
thirty
answ
abdo
the b
nurs
Pete
saic
mig

sta
en
by
ta
o
a
e

which he had to swallow a thin liquid called gastrographin rather than the usual thicker barium (due to the risk of vomiting and then aspirating barium into his lungs). Although gastrographin shows the outline of a structure or obstruction, it may not show details of the stomach lining or small intestine and may also miss spasm or irregularities, especially at the junction of surgical incisions in the intestine.

By now, every time Peter swallowed, he regurgitated. He was told that this must be the result of diabetic gastroparesis, in which the stomach does not empty, and that there was medically nothing to be done. That day, a surgeon appeared, introduced himself, reviewed the various imaging results, and told Peter that because of the gastric stapling and resulting anatomic changes, he was not a candidate for any surgical procedure except the placement of a feeding tube in his small intestine.

Peter finally saw a family practitioner, who explained that because there was no medical treatment for his condition, he should be discharged that day and follow a liquid diet. If he became dehydrated or vomited, he should return to the ER, and it might be necessary to put in a feeding tube. This would mean he could not taste or swallow food and would need to ingest an emulsified substance through the tube throughout the day. Peter asked whether a specialist for this kind of problem could see him before he was discharged, and the doctor responded that she'd had prior experience in a similar case. Reluctantly, she agreed to call in a gastroenterologist, who could not see him until the next day.

The next morning, Peter was woken by the gastroenterologist. She took another brief history, did another brief physical exam, and told Peter that after she'd reviewed his x-rays and scans, she would return to advise him. She didn't come back until the end of the day, and said that she fully agreed with the family practitioner's recommendation. Although an experimental drug was being used in Europe for this problem, it was not legally available in the United States, so she felt that the advice to go home and "wait it out" was the appropriate management.

Peter was stunned, confused, angry, and frightened. Each day in the hospital, he'd continued to have multiple vomiting episodes; he was in the dark as to what was being done or what he was being given; and there appeared to be significant dissociation between the various doctors, nurses, and orderlies. At this point, Peter called another doctor's office, as they were socially acquainted, and told the whole story. The doctor thought an upper endoscopy should be performed to determine whether any severe acid reflux was causing an undetected esophageal narrowing or whether there was a narrowing of the junction between the esophagus and stomach, between the stomach and small intestine, or at the site of the gastric stapling.

After multiple phone calls, the doctor finally reached the gastroenterologist and urged her to do an upper endoscopy to assess the esophageal and stomach lining for any strictures or inflammation that could be contributing to Peter's symptoms. She assured him that this was unnecessary because she had performed a motility study, and the general impression was that he had a "motility disorder." Furthermore, Peter had undergone an upper endoscopy because of heartburn four months previously, and it had been totally normal. The doctor pointed out that this was many weeks before the onset of his current difficulty, but she responded that repeating the procedure was clearly not cost-effective.

The doctor then called the hospital's chief of gastroenterology. Although he did not think that it was cost-effective or would be covered, in deference to this doctor, he agreed to urge the gastroenterologist to reconsider an upper endoscopy, which was reluctantly performed the next day. The esophageal and stomach lining were reported to look fine, but as the endoscope approached the site of the gastric stapling, there seemed to be an area of narrowing. When the endoscope was pushed through, it easily dilated the relative narrowing, but the gastroenterologist did not think this was "clinically significant."

Peter was discharged that afternoon, still ingesting only liquids. Once or twice a day thereafter, the doctor spoke with him by phone about everything he consumed. They started with liquids, then puddings, and then moved to soft foods and eventually to solid foods. After that endoscopy, he had no subsequent swallowing difficulty, regurgitation, or vomiting. Like so many others, Peter had been the victim of a dysfunctional healthcare system.

By contrast, consider Richard, a fifty-eight-year-old businessman in a concierge medicine program. He had diabetes and reported frequent heartburn but was noncompliant with treatment. He forgot to take the prescribed medication, refused to give up alcohol, and did not regularly follow dietary precautions. When he called with a feeling of fullness and vague abdominal discomfort, an outpatient upper endoscopy was performed the next day. The expected signs of esophageal reflux irritation were not present, but a large mass was found at the far end of the stomach, and multiple biopsies showed cancer of the stomach.

The next day, Richard was seen by an oncologist and a stomach surgeon, and the following day by another oncologist and another surgeon for second opinions. All of the consultants agreed that surgery was necessary because of likely complete obstruction in the near future. Because Richard's diabetes had been poorly controlled and he was found to be anemic, it was decided to bring him into the hospital twenty-four hours before the planned surgery to regulate his blood sugar and begin blood transfusions.

On the day of admission, he was met at the information desk by one of the patient coordinators and escorted to a private room. An admissions officer came to the room to obtain his signature on the hospital forms. Richard had been able to review them in advance, and the office had already submitted his insurance information, so the entire admission procedure took less than five minutes. The floor nurse then came in to take his vital signs. His blood was drawn, typed, and cross-matched in preparation for the transfusions.

After breakfast, Richard was seen by a diabetologist who advised him on the management of his diabetes. About midday, he received his first transfusion. An EKG (electrocardiogram) that morning had revealed an irregularity in his heart rhythm, so a cardiologist saw him shortly after lunch, giving clearance for anesthesia and recommending treatment for his rhythm change. The oncologist visited and reviewed the prior findings and recommendations for post-operative treatment. Then the surgeon came in and did a complete physical exam, reviewed the planned operation, and asked

Richard to sign consent forms for surgery and anesthesia. That night, a "Do Not Disturb" sign was placed on his door, the door was closed, and he had a good night's sleep.

Richard was the first patient on the surgical schedule the following morning and underwent an uncomplicated operation. Throughout his hospitalization, his doctor saw him twice a day and was completely informed of everything performed and planned. The doctor could ensure that all administered drugs were appropriate, that tests were done expeditiously, that he was not left waiting around in cold hallways, that vital signs were not taken unnecessarily while he was resting, and that his privacy was protected. At discharge four days after the surgery, his medications were delivered with explanations, and he was escorted to his car without delay. Four weeks later, he was free of discomfort and working as hard as ever.

As you can see, these two patients had two very different hospitalization experiences. This section addresses many of the potential battles of hospital care.

 ## ARE THERE RELIABLE WEB SITES WITH ACCURATE INFORMATION ON THE QUALITY OF HOSPITALS IN MY AREA?

Yes. Here are four such Web sites: the *US News & World Report* ranking of American hospitals is available at www.usnews.com/usnews/health;

hospital ratings by performance, diagnosis, and treatment are at www.healthgrade.com; quality assessments by the Joint Commission (an organization that accredits healthcare facilities) are at www.qualitycheck.org; and assessments of hospitals with regard to outcomes of heart attacks, heart failure, and pneumonia can be found at www.hospitalcompare.hhs.gov.

 ### IF I GO TO A TEACHING HOSPITAL, WILL I BE A GUINEA PIG?

No. In a teaching hospital, you will receive care from physicians at all levels of training as well as from their supervising licensed physicians. It may be tedious to undergo evaluations by a medical student, intern, resident, one or more subspecialty fellows, and the attending physician, but there is a benefit to multiple histories and multiple physicals— you never know which doctor will detect something that will make all the difference. And in times of crisis or emergency, having many physicians available around the clock is a great advantage. There are also disadvantages, as mistakes can be made, but the many layers of supervision are designed to avoid mistakes.

Another distinct advantage of most teaching hospitals is that they can provide state-of-the-art diagnosis and treatment in most areas of medicine.

The attending physicians are usually highly respected and well-qualified. The same can be said of many community, county, and veterans' administration hospitals as well. Of course, some provide excellent care and some do not. In many states, a Web site provides information about objective measures of quality at various hospitals.

At a teaching hospital, you may be approached to participate in a clinical trial. If so, you should be fully informed of both the upside and downside of participating. You should not feel obligated to participate. At no time should you be included in any experimental or clinical trial without your written consent. (There is an exception to this when you are incapacitated, and the person authorized to make decisions for you decides that you should have an experimental treatment.) A wise patient will not agree to participate without consulting his or her attending physician about the potential benefits and the potential risks.

 HOW DO I KNOW WHETHER THE HOSPITAL I'M BEING REFERRED TO IS A GOOD PLACE FOR THE PARTICULAR PROCEDURE I NEED?

There is no doubt that the best results are achieved at medical institutions with the broadest experience. A hospital that performs 300 liver transplants a year, for instance, is likely to have better outcomes with this surgery than a hospital that performs ten per year. Often there is a dramatic difference between results at a small local hospital and results at a major medical center. Whether your intended hospital is large or small, be sure it is accredited by the Joint Commission (formerly known as the JCAHO).

Seek evidence that your assigned surgeon and anesthesiologist both have vast experience with the procedure. For example, it has been recommended that for open-heart surgery, you should utilize a hospital that does at least 500 of these operations per year; for carotid artery surgery, 100 per year; for esophagectomy, 13 per year; for mastectomy, 25 per year; for pediatric heart surgery, 100 per year; for prostate surgery, 55 per year; and for repair of abdominal aortic aneurysms, 30 per year. To obtain this kind of information, check with the office of the hospital director.

 HOW DO I KNOW WHETHER THE RECOMMENDED SURGEON IS REALLY A GOOD SURGEON?

See the question and answer in Section Two about finding a good doctor. In addition, talk to an anesthesiologist, other doctors, and a nurse in the hospital about who they would use for this surgery. These kinds of recommendations may not be infallible, but they certainly may help.

## ARE THERE ANY TIPS ON WHEN I SHOULD SCHEDULE ELECTIVE HOSPITALIZATION?

If you are planning a non-urgent procedure at a university-affiliated hospital, it is often wise to try to avoid having it during the first months of the training year. Most interns, residents, and fellows begin their training year on July 1, so July can be an especially difficult month at a hospital. Faculty at most academic institutions are especially involved during the summer to ensure continued quality of care—but if you can avoid a July or August admission, you may avoid potential problems.

Staffing on weekends and holidays may not be as extensive as it is during the regular workweek. Most hospitals can handle urgent problems at any time, but a wise patient tries to avoid scheduling elective procedures for times when hospital staffing may be less than optimal.

 ## HOW DO I EXPEDITE MY ADMISSIONS PROCESS?

Hospitals commonly instruct all incoming patients to arrive at the admissions office at about the same time in the morning. Then, usually on a first-come-first-served basis, an admissions officer meets with each waiting patient and provides a series of forms. After the forms are signed and insurance information is obtained, the patient waits to be escorted to a hospital room. The best thing you can do to influence this process is to ask your physician (or an administrator or nurse at your physician's office) to call the hospital's admissions office on your behalf and request expedited processing. This may not always work, but it is worth a try.

If you participate in a concierge medicine program, much of the waiting is eliminated. A patient coordinator meets you at the admissions office to facilitate, assist with forms, and transport you expeditiously to your hospital room.

 HOW DO I GET INTO A HOSPITAL ROOM WHEN "ALL THE BEDS ARE FILLED"?

This is becoming a very common problem. Some parts of the United States have too many urgent-care patients and not enough hospital rooms. In most instances when a hospital is filled, your options are to use a different hospital (if your admitting physician has admitting privileges elsewhere), to wait until a room becomes available, or to get your doctor involved in facilitating the availability of a bed.

Let me give you an example. A concerned wife called her doctor one morning because her husband had been running a fever throughout the night, and when she awoke she'd found him in their bedroom closet, disoriented and coughing heavily. The doctor agreed to meet them at the emergency room, called ahead to reserve an ER bed, and called a pulmonologist in their concierge network. They both evaluated the patient at the ER. He had a temperature of 103°F, his chest x-ray showed extensive pneumonia, and he needed to be admitted to the hospital for intravenous antibiotics, heart monitoring, and blood gas evaluations. However, the hospital was filled. They could continue his care in the ER in the hope that a bed would eventually become available, or they could try to manipulate the system.

The doctor called the hospital's bed control office and learned that no other seriously ill patients in the ER or elsewhere required admission. He then spoke with the charge nurse on the private room floor who told him about two patients who might be discharged that day, including one in a monitored bed. He knew that patient's attending physician, so when he called him at home, he agreed to come into the hospital to reevaluate his patient, and discharge orders were subsequently written. The staff was very cooperative in expediting that patient's discharge and cleaning the room quickly. Within an hour, the patient was moved from the ER to a private room with a monitored bed, when earlier that day "all beds were filled."

The message here is that some extra time and effort on the part of your physician can really pay off. In this situation, a very sick patient's needs were met efficiently without adversely affecting any other patient.

## HOW CAN I GET A PRIVATE ROOM WHEN I'M TOLD THAT NONE ARE AVAILABLE?

If you participate in a concierge medicine program, or if your family doctor or a member of your doctor's staff is willing, a call to the hospital's bed control office or nursing services administration on your behalf may be helpful in obtaining a private room. That day's planned discharges can be reviewed, and sometimes a patient's discharge can be expedited to make a private room available for a new admission.

## WHO ARE ALL THE DIFFERENT DOCTORS I MAY BE SEEING?

Any number of physicians may meet with you during your hospitalization. At smaller hospitals, you are likely to be seen only by your own doctor or designated surgeon. At larger teaching hospitals, an attending physician is in charge of your care, and several kinds of in-house physicians report to the attending physician. An intern has received the doctor of medicine degree and is in the first year of training after medical school. A resident has completed an internship and is in three to seven years of training for board certification in a specialty such as internal medicine or surgery. A fellow has completed internship and residency and is a state-licensed physician in training to become a subspecialist such as a gastroenterologist, cardiologist, or orthopedic surgeon.

At a private or community hospital, you may be seen by a doctor who is covering for your doctor. In addition, consultants in relevant specialties and subspecialties may be asked to take a history, do a physical exam, and make recommendations about your diagnosis and treatment. At a university hospital or a university-affiliated teaching hospital, a medical student may take a history and perform a physical exam, an intern and a resident may do the same, and the attending physician will have already heard reports from each of the other physicians before he or she evaluates you.

You may be annoyed by repetitive examinations and questions, but it is often in the patient's best interest to have several minds thinking about the medical problems at hand. It is not unusual for a physician in training to detect important features in the patient's history that give a clue to an unsuspected diagnosis. Although inexperienced physicians may make mistakes, in most instances their supervision is close enough that the benefit outweighs any risk. There is also a great advantage in the constant availability of physicians at a teaching hospital to manage situations that develop at odd hours. Although some private hospitals have several physicians present around the clock, that is quite unusual.

## WHO ARE ALL THE DIFFERENT NURSES?

In many institutions, nurses wear a name badge indicating whether they are an RN (registered nurse) or an LVN (licensed vocational nurse). An RN has completed nursing school, has a nursing degree, and is allowed to administer narcotics and IV drugs as well as all routine medications. An LVN has completed a shorter period of training and assists in routine nursing activities such as taking vital signs but is not allowed to administer narcotics or IV drugs. A care partner is an assistant who has limited training but may help lift patients, assist them in walking, sit in the room to be available for assistance in getting out of bed, or provide other backup support of this nature to the regular nursing staff.

A charge nurse is in charge of a nursing unit and oversees the quality of nursing care in the patient rooms surrounding a given nursing station. A nursing supervisor oversees the quality of nursing care in all or part of the medical center or institution. Nursing supervisors are often troubleshooters and are in charge of allocating nursing care to the areas of greatest need.

## WHILE I'M HOSPITALIZED, WHAT SHOULD I DO TO MAINTAIN GOOD RELATIONSHIPS WITH THE STAFF?

Be nice and cooperative while you are inquisitive and questioning. Be an advocate for your own needs but in a friendly and non-confrontational manner. Keep a dish of candy in your room for the staff. Order a pizza or a basket of cookies or muffins for the nurse's station. Say "thank you" and "please" and treat all staff with respect. After you are discharged, write a letter to the hospital's CEO that describes what you liked about the staff and the care you received.

## HOW DO I GET HOSPITAL PERSONNEL TO PAY MORE ATTENTION TO ME?

Most people respond to respect, kindness, and thoughtfulness, and it is generally wise to take that approach before becoming confrontational or angry. If you try that but still feel that staff members are treating you more as a number than as a person, it is perfectly appropriate to point this out in a friendly way.

If you wish, you can send the staff a cake, flowers, or a box of cookies or candy to thank them for their services and kindnesses. They will remember you warmly and personally in the future.

## HOW SHOULD I HANDLE A CRANKY OR ALOOF NURSE OR OTHER STAFF MEMBER?

No patient should be subjected to disrespect, inefficiency, or rudeness. However, staff members at hospitals and doctors' offices are often under intense pressure and may be overworked and underpaid. This does not excuse poor performance or bad attitudes, but it can provide some level of understanding.

When a staff member is unfriendly, uncooperative, or insulting, first "kill them with love." It is very difficult for a person to continue being rude to a friendly, cordial, and cheerful patient. If this approach does not work, gently asking why he or she is being rude or unfriendly may cause the staff member to think twice. If this does not work, speak with the supervisor. Most supervisors respond to a reasonable complaint by counseling or reassigning the staff member and facilitating excellent service to the patient. If all else has failed, ask your physician to discuss the situation with the hospital's senior staff.

## SHOULD I TAKE EVERY PILL AND UNDERGO EVERY TEST AS DIRECTED BY THE NURSES AND ORDERLIES?

A nurse should identify any medications administered and describe why they are being given. Ask for that information if it is not offered, and if it does not make sense, call your doctor for clarification, or ask the nurse to double-check to be sure that an error is not being made. When an orderly arrives to take you for testing, ask about the nature of the test. If the doctor has not already explained the test to you and indicated that it would be done, call the doctor, or ask the staff to double-check to be sure that test has indeed been ordered for you.

 I'VE HEARD HORROR STORIES ABOUT PEOPLE HAVING THE WRONG LEG OR THE WRONG SIDE OF THE BODY OPERATED ON. HOW DO I AVOID BEING A VICTIM OF HOSPITAL ERROR?

Such events are quite rare, but for certainty and your own peace of mind, ask your doctor to use a marker to indicate "yes" and "no" on the appropriate limbs or sides. (Many surgeons do this routinely.) To help prevent medication errors, be sure you know what drugs have been prescribed for you, and keep a list of the drugs that you're taking. When a nurse brings you any medication, ask what it is, what it is for, and what the dosage is. The better hospitals have a history of fewer errors; you can check out your hospital's record at www.hospitalcompare.hhs.gov and www.healthgrades.com.

Good things as well as bad things happen in hospitals. Weekends and holidays can be dangerous, as a full crew may not be present. Mistakes seem to be more common at night, when patients may be less closely observed (except, of course, in the intensive care unit). Night staff members are often reluctant to awaken senior physicians and tend to try to handle problems until they become serious and more difficult to treat. Hospital staff members also work long hours, and fatigue may contribute to errors and poor judgment.

Let me illustrate with a patient's story. Robert is sixty-one years old and obese, has a long history of anxiety, and takes a variety of antidepressants. He also has a history of heart disease and has developed type II diabetes. When he saw blood in his urine, urologic tests showed a large tumor of the left kidney. He was not a candidate for laparoscopic surgery, instead he required open surgery under general anesthesia. This meant that a week prior to his scheduled admission, he would need to discontinue the anticoagulant he had been taking. For obvious reasons, Robert was considered a very high-risk patient, so his doctor substituted a short-acting anticoagulant as a precaution prior to surgery.

After the successful surgery, Robert's internist, concerned about the risk of post-operative heart attack or stroke, wrote a note each day requesting that anticoagulation be reinstituted. The urologist and his team, however, thought this would be unsafe because of the potential for bleeding at the site of the surgery, so anticoagulation was not reinstituted. Robert was slated for discharge about a week after surgery. The day prior to the scheduled discharge, the internist again wrote a note urging that if the patient was healthy enough to be discharged, he was healthy enough to have anticoagulation.

That night, Robert developed constricting, severe chest pain. An EKG revealed evidence of a heart attack, which was confirmed by a blood test, and emergency angiography was promptly performed. Two partially occluded blood vessels had to be propped open with stents. Robert then spent four days in intensive care and another three days on the cardiac observation floor. Fortunately, he survived his post-operative heart attack. Could it have been prevented? Were there mistakes in judgment? These questions are difficult to answer.

 ### HOW DO I REDUCE THE AMOUNT OF TIME I SPEND IN THE HOSPITAL FOR TESTING?

Discuss this with the doctor in charge of your care, and ask for tests to be scheduled at a rate that is comfortable for you. You may feel, for instance, that you do not want to be stressed or subjected to multiple tests in a short time period without enough rest. Alternatively, you may feel that you would like as many of your tests as possible to be scheduled within a day, to facilitate an earlier diagnosis, treatment, and discharge. If you participate in a concierge medicine program, your physician or his or her staff should expedite your testing according to your preferences.

 ## HOW DO I GET PRIVACY IN THE HOSPITAL?

Fortunately, there is currently a renewed effort within the medical profession to protect the privacy of patient information and respect the privacy needs of individuals. Unfortunately, some hospital staff members forget the importance of patient privacy.

A private room is the first step, if one is available and you can afford it. If you are sharing a room, wear a bathrobe and slippers (you may need to bring these from home). If you must wear a standard hospital gown, consider requesting two gowns, so you can wear one tied in back and one tied in front and be more completely covered. Keeping the curtains drawn around your bed may be helpful but also may be confining.

Do not be afraid to be your own advocate in protecting your privacy. If a doctor or a nurse starts to expose you in front of others, ask him or her to do so privately. If people tend to enter your room without knocking, place a note on the door requesting a knock before entering. If nurses enter your room throughout the night and this makes you uncomfortable, ask your doctor whether this is really necessary.

## HOW DO I GET SOME SLEEP IN THE HOSPITAL?

Hospitals are typically busy and noisy around the clock. You are likely to get more rest in a private room. In any room, ask that your door be kept closed. Place a sign on the door indicating that you are sleeping and asking that the door be opened quietly. Ask your doctor whether it is really necessary for your vital signs to be taken during the night. Because "routine" orders are often written at admission, nighttime vital signs may be ordered for patients who turn out to be stable enough not to require them, so a second look at this issue may get you more privacy and more rest. You can also ask whether medications administered during the night could be given to you during waking hours instead.

 ## HOW DO I GET RESPECT IN THE HOSPITAL?

As in all areas of life, there are always some people who treat others with apparent disrespect. In a medical situation, this often occurs inadvertently. Many people, for example, find it offensive for a stranger such as a covering doctor, a nurse, or an orderly to address them by their first name. However, some people prefer it. You need to indicate your own preferences. If a staff member addresses you as Mr., Mrs., or Ms., but you'd like to be called by your first name, just say so. On the other hand, if you aren't comfortable with that level of familiarity, you may get the message across simply by treating others as you would like to be treated—that is, address the orderly, nurse, or new doctor as Mr., Ms., or Doctor so-and-so. If they don't catch on, there is really nothing wrong with saying that you're more comfortable being addressed as Mr., Mrs., or Ms. until you know each other better and then get on a first-name basis.

 ### IF I HAVE A COMPLAINT WHEN I'M IN THE HOSPITAL, WHOM SHOULD I SPEAK TO?

Talk to the doctor in charge of your care, as he or she should be your advocate. If you do not want to go to that level, talk to the nurse; if that does not make a difference, complain to the charge nurse; and if that fails, ask for the nursing supervisor. Use common sense—the seriousness of the issue should decide how high you go to make your complaint known. Every hospital has a chief executive officer whose office receives complaints and usually responds.

 ### HOW DO I GET A GOOD PRIVATE DUTY NURSE IN THE HOSPITAL?

Most private duty nurses are represented by professional registries. Ask your friends whether they can recommend nurses that they have used, or ask the charge nurse on your hospital floor to recommend a private nurse. Some hospital nurses do private duty nursing when they aren't working in the hospital. If you participate in a concierge medicine program, your doctor's staff probably works with a group of private nurses who they can recommend and/or call on your behalf.

# SECTION 6
## A Short Primer on Drugs

Marvin reported having heartburn more than three times a week, so his doctor advised him to avoid alcohol, caffeine, and peppermint—peppermint weakens the lower esophageal sphincter and allows acid reflux up from the stomach. He was also advised to take an acid-reducing medication from a modern group of drugs called PPIs (proton pump inhibitors). At a dose of one 40-milligram tablet daily, his symptoms persisted, so his doctor increased the dose to one tablet at breakfast and one at dinner, and this did the trick. All of Marvin's symptoms went away within a few days.

Because Marvin was now taking two tablets a day as instructed, his bottle of pills rapidly emptied. His doctor had prescribed three refills, but when Marvin went to a local pharmacy to obtain more medication, the pharmacist told him his insurance company would not approve the medication because the initial prescription for a one-month supply at one tablet per day meant that Marvin was not due for a refill for several days. To hold him over, the pharmacist offered to sell him additional pills at a cost of approximately $12 each.

Fortunately, Marvin had several other options. He could call his physician and ask for a revised prescription to obtain the currently prescribed dosage under his insurance coverage. Alternatively, he could ask the pharmacist whether there was any generic form of the prescribed medication that would be less expensive. He could also ask his physician or pharmacist whether there was an over-the-counter medication equivalent to the prescribed drug—and in this case, there was. Omeprazole is an over-the-counter PPI available in 10- or 20-milligram tablets at a fraction of the cost of the prescription PPI. To ensure comparable relief, the patient may have to take two pills instead of one, but the cost savings can be significant.

Drugs may have side effects, are often expensive, and may interact with other drugs (or foods) with a resulting decrease or increase in their potency. This section provides some basic information that you should know about any medications you may take.

## WHY DO DRUGS HAVE TWO NAMES?

Most drugs have a brand name for marketing as well as a chemical name that describes their chemical composition. An example is the drug with the brand name Imuran and the chemical name 6-mercaptopurine; another is aspirin, with the chemical name acetylsalicylic acid. If a drug is produced and marketed by more than one manufacturer, its brand names will differ, but chemical names remain the same regardless of the manufacturer or whether it's a brand-name or generic drug.

 ## WHAT DOES IT MEAN WHEN A DRUG "GOES GENERIC"?

The federal government allows pharmaceutical companies to obtain a patent that protects a newly developed drug from being copied by other pharmaceutical companies in the United States for seventeen years. During this period of exclusive rights to manufacture the drug and oversee its distribution, the company tries to recoup its development costs and make a profit. After the patent period, any pharmaceutical company with proper capabilities can copy, sell, and distribute the drug. At that point, marketplace competition often results in a dramatic price reduction. The drug may be sold under different brand names and may also be available as a generic drug without a brand name.

## SHOULD I USE GENERIC DRUGS OR STICK TO BRAND NAMES?

If you insist on a brand-name medication over its generic counterpart, you may pay a premium price. Ask your doctor whether there is any reason not to use a generic version of your medication if it is available. Generic drugs manufactured in the United States are produced under FDA guidelines and supervision and are generally equivalent to brand-name drugs. The financial savings in using generic medications can be significant.

Be cautious, however, about obtaining either brand-name or generic drugs on the Internet or from foreign countries. Drugs produced outside of the United States do not have FDA surveillance, and you cannot be certain of their equivalent potency or safety. Some Internet vendors profiteer by selling marginal or less-effective medications, and counterfeit drugs are rampant. However, you may find a reputable foreign pharmacist or an Internet vendor with a stamp of approval by the National Association of Boards of Pharmacy or designation as a VIPPS (Verified Internet Pharmacy Practice Site.

## HOW ELSE CAN I REDUCE THE COST OF MY MEDICATIONS?

Be an alert consumer. Some pharmaceutical companies charge approximately the same amount of money per pill regardless of the dosage contained in the pill. You may find, for example, that some pharmacies sell a particular 10-milligram pill for as much money as a 40-milligram pill of the same medication. In such a case, if you need a 40-milligram dose, be sure to order the 40-milligram pill specifically rather than four 10-milligram pills.

Low-income patients may wish to take advantage of the drug discount cards offered by most major pharmaceutical companies. And if you are a senior citizen, most drugstores will give you a senior discount if you ask.

 ### WHAT'S THE DIFFERENCE BETWEEN A DRUG ALLERGY AND A DRUG SIDE EFFECT?

An allergy is an immunological reaction to a foreign substance such as a drug. If your immune system responds to exposure to a drug by developing antibodies against it, these antibodies then interact with the drug when you take it, and the result may be an allergic reaction of itching, rash, asthma, swelling of the larynx and/or lips, difficulty breathing, or various other symptoms.

A side effect is also an adverse response to a drug, but it does not involve the development of antibodies and may evolve over a longer time period while taking the medication. Most drugs have some side effects that typically affect some people, although many drugs approved by the FDA (Food and Drug Administration) only produce side effects in a small percentage of people. Common side effects are nausea, diarrhea, constipation, muscle aches, and many others—some serious, some not so serious.

Whether you experience an allergic reaction or a problematic side effect in response to a medication, notify your doctor promptly. The drug you're taking will probably need to be substituted with another drug in a different family of pharmaceuticals.

 ### WHY ARE SO MANY DOCTORS SO NEGATIVE ABOUT ALTERNATIVE MEDI-CINE?

The term "alternative medicine" encompasses a vast array of herbal and other remedies as well as treatments including acupuncture, therapeutic massage, meditation, homeopathy, aromatherapy, and many more. Some people benefit from alternative medicine, and some people do not.

The negativism among many physicians toward much of alternative medicine reflects the general lack of objective, scientifically obtained supporting data. The traditional premise of medicine is, "First do no harm." As most alternative treatments have not been subjected to prospective, controlled clinical trials, it is difficult to determine whether they are harmful or helpful. Many people are nevertheless convinced of these treatments' efficacy and safety.

Many doctors and some medical schools are currently integrating conventional and alternative medicine in treatment planning.

The major pharmaceutical companies that have substantial research budgets and fund most clinical trials do not produce alternative medicines. It would undoubtedly benefit our healthcare system, however, to find funding for well-designed clinical trials of alternative treatments to determine what works (and why) and what does not—as well as what is safe and what is not.

##  ARE HERBAL SUPPLEMENTS AND FDA-APPROVED DRUGS EQUALLY SAFE?

Before a pharmaceutical company can market a medication, the newly developed drug is first subjected to extensive laboratory and animal testing before it is ever administered to a human being. Then it must be tested in thousands of patients in well-controlled, prospective clinical trials that follow the participants for long periods of time to determine the drug's safety and effectiveness. A large amount of data must be submitted for review by FDA staff and an additional committee of experts to obtain FDA approval. After the drug is FDA-approved, it can be marketed. The company is required to continue reporting any adverse reactions to that drug, as some side effects may not become apparent until the drug is utilized in even larger patient populations over a longer period of time.

In comparison, an herbal supplement is classified as a food additive, and the FDA does not evaluate food additives. Stores can therefore sell herbal supplements produced without any governmental supervision and without any data supporting manufacturers' claims of safety and effectiveness. Ingredients may differ from batch to batch, and there may be contaminants. The presence of a product in a drugstore does not necessarily mean that it is safe.

The bottom line is that FDA-approved drugs are subjected to extensive testing and regulation, whereas herbal products are not. When an herbal supplement is marked "USP-verified," this indicates that the United States Pharmacopeia, a nonprofit scientific organization, has verified that the supplement contains what the label says it contains. USP verification does not guarantee, however, that the supplement is either effective or safe.

 I'VE SEEN ADS FOR A PRESCRIPTION DRUG THAT I'M INTERESTED IN TAKING. SHOULD I TELL MY DOCTOR ABOUT IT?

Last year, people in the United States consumed $279 billion worth of prescription medications. And last year, the world's pharmaceutical companies spent an estimated $19

billion on marketing to convince patients and doctors to utilize brand-name drugs—even though three-quarters of all prescription drugs in the United States are available as cheaper generics. Marketing turns patients and physicians toward new drugs with side effects and risks that are not very well known, and away from older, cheaper, equally effective drugs with a longer history of use and safety. As more doctors prescribe the newest brand-name drugs, medication costs increase.

There is nothing wrong with marketing new drugs if they are safe, effective, and priced competitively. However, financial incentives can lead to inappropriate risks and may raise the cost of healthcare. Sometimes physicians rely too heavily on information provided by drug company representatives. The pharmaceutical industry counters such criticism by pointing out that it costs tens of millions of dollars to bring a single new drug to market from the beginning of development to final FDA approval; that the industry's sponsorship of research on new drugs may significantly benefit innumerable patients; and that marketing to physicians provides busy clinicians with valuable information for their treatment decisions. So the debate over the pros and cons of drug marketing goes on.

Direct television advertising to the healthcare consumer has greatly increased in recent years, including promotions for prescription drugs that can be used to lower cholesterol, reduce acid reflux, and counteract numerous other health problems. When you discuss your symptoms and conditions with your doctor, there is no harm in mentioning advertisements for medications of possible interest. For me, however, the bottom line is that physicians, rather than patients, are best trained to assess a drug's safety and effectiveness.

Physicians know how to evaluate promotions and scientific reports and also have experience with the use of various drugs. Most patients do not have a background that enables them to make these judgments. The final decision about the appropriateness of any drug should be made by a well-trained physician.

# SECTION 7
## Healthcare While Traveling

Richard, a middle-aged businessman visiting Los Angeles, slipped and fell in the shower in his hotel room. He hit his head on the floor but did not lose consciousness. Afterward, he had a bruise on his forehead, and his wife was concerned, though he protested that he felt fine. She called their concierge doctor in New York and reached the doctor covering the service for the weekend. He called a cooperating Los Angeles office and was put through to one of the associates, as the offices had an agreement to care for each other's concierge patients in their respective cities.

The associate went to the hotel, examined Richard, and found no abnormalities other than the bruise. Nevertheless, he then escorted Richard to the emergency room, after calling ahead to ensure an examining room and alert the radiologist. Richard was rapidly evaluated in the ER and taken promptly for a head CT scan; everything was found to be normal. He left the ER in less than ninety minutes and was very grateful for his thorough care. Communication with his own doctor made a big difference in getting good care rapidly and effectively, even though he was traveling.

Health problems can be especially difficult when you're traveling. This section provides some helpful advice that should make your travel health issues easier to manage.

 ### HOW CAN I BE SURE TO GET GOOD HEALTHCARE IF I'M SICK OR INJURED WHEN TRAVELING?

When you are traveling within the United States and become ill or sustain an injury, it is usually a good idea to call your doctor in your own city. He or she may be able to identify a colleague in your location or at least speak to a physician on your behalf. If you are taken to an ER for urgent treatment, a phone call from your doctor back home may expedite your care. It's generally a safe bet that a university hospital wherever you are has well-qualified physicians on its faculty. Most hotels also have physicians on call.

If you participate in a concierge medicine program, your doctor may be affiliated with a network of doctors in other communities in the United States and even in foreign countries. Accordingly, a call to your concierge doctor may guide you in the right direction.

It is especially helpful when traveling to be prepared with a list of your medications and their dosages, any current conditions, and a chronological history of your prior illnesses.

 ### IF I NEED A DOCTOR OR AM BROUGHT TO AN EMERGENCY ROOM IN A FOREIGN CITY, WHOM CAN I TRUST?

If you find yourself in need of healthcare when you're out of the country, the same principles apply as in the item above. You would be wise to call your family doctor and ask him or her to speak directly to the doctor or ER director on your behalf. Even internationally, doctor-to-doctor contact can go a long way in getting you good care. Some hospitals provide translators. Nevertheless, if you can involve (or bring along) a friend or relative who speaks the language of the country you're visiting, your healthcare issue may be easier to handle.

 ### WHEN I'M TRAVELING, CAN I TRUST FOREIGN DRUGS?

Yes and no. Many pharmaceuticals made in foreign countries are safe and effective, but some are not. Find a physician in the foreign community through one of the routes described above, and seek his or her advice or assistance in obtaining safe and effective medication.

WHAT SHOULD I DO IF I RUN OUT OF MY MEDICATIONS WHILE I'M TRAVELING?

If you have any health conditions or are currently taking any prescribed medication, carry with you a written prescription for anything that you might need while traveling. Prescriptions are generally honored nationwide across the United States and at most foreign pharmacies as well. It may be helpful to get the number of a local pharmacy near your hotel, call your doctor back home, and ask him or her to call the pharmacy and prescribe the medication refill for you directly.

 I'M CONCERNED THAT WHEN I TRAVEL INTERNATIONALLY, MY MEDICATIONS MAY CAUSE A PROBLEM IF MY BAGS ARE INSPECTED. HOW SHOULD I HANDLE THIS?

Only take medications into or out of other countries in the original pharmacy containers. It is wise to carry a copy of each of your prescriptions to document your need for the medications you're carrying. Another good idea is to ask your physician to give you a note on his or her professional letterhead, listing each of your medications and the doses and providing his or her DEA (Drug Enforcement Administration) number and medical license number. If you must carry any narcotic, it is imperative to carry a copy of the original prescription as well as a letter from your physician containing the information just described. If you purchase any drugs that are not allowed in the United States, do not bring them back with you.

## ARE CRUISE-SHIP DOCTORS RELIABLE?

Yes and no. If you're planning a cruise, inquire about the background of the doctor on the ship. Some of these doctors are in training, and even though they may be competent subspecialty fellows or medical residents, they may lack the experience of a more seasoned general physician. Other cruise-ship doctors may be semi-retired or retired physicians who trained in a subspecialty, but for the purpose of the cruise, are practicing general medicine—not always a good idea.

In one incident, a woman became ill on a trip and visited the cruise-ship doctor, who had to pull out a medical textbook to look up the treatment for her symptoms. If you find yourself in such a situation, you need to be your own advocate. You may wish to call your own doctor back home to discuss your symptoms and the treatment provided, and he or she may be able to talk directly to the cruise-ship doctor to facilitate your care.

### WHEN I TRAVEL, SHOULD I BUY MEDICAL EVACUATION INSURANCE AND TRAVEL HEALTH INSURANCE?

Both are good ideas, if you can afford them—the premiums can be quite high. The policies, however, may have specific limitations to certain areas or certain conditions or may require that the justification for a medical evacuation meet the insurance company's criteria, which may not be same as your criteria. Accordingly, be sure to read your policy carefully before leaving on your trip.

### HOW DO I AVOID TRAVELER'S DIARRHEA?

Traveler's diarrhea is usually due to an infection transmitted by water, raw fruits and vegetables, and sometimes even the knives that are used to cut raw produce. Your physician should be able to tell you where traveler's diarrhea is prevalent. In these areas, drink only bottled water or canned or bottled beverages, brush your teeth with bottled water, and avoid adding ice cubes to your drinks. As a rule of thumb, you can safely eat fruits and vegetables that need to be peeled but not cut. Eating produce that needs to be washed and cut is risky. Your physician may suggest an antibiotic to prevent traveler's diarrhea, and may prescribe an antibiotic if diarrhea does develop.

## HOW DO I AVOID DVT ON LONG FLIGHTS?

DVT (deep venous thrombosis) is a blood clot, often with associated inflammation, in a vein in either or both legs. This can be a very serious health problem. Such a clot may be dislodged and go to your lung, causing a pulmonary embolism (destruction of lung tissue), or travel to your brain and cause a stroke. Long flights can lead to pooling of blood in the legs, which makes it easier for clots to form. As a precautionary measure against DVT, it is a good idea to get out of your seat and walk the length of the plane once or twice on an hourly basis. In addition, avoid crossing your legs while you're sitting for any long period of time.

# EPILOGUE

The first part of this book has dealt with how to care for yourself, how to use common sense to improve the quality of your current life and quality of life as you age. It stresses the importance of a healthy lifestyle in order to improve the likelihood of successful aging. Rather than living long and miserably, we should all strive to live long and enjoyably. Taking personal responsibility for our health and well-being is the key to getting well. Staying well also requires a common-sense approach to diet, nutrition, exercise and meditation. Currently more is needed.

While the healthcare system remains dysfunctional, one must advocate on one's own behalf or one must find someone to serve as an advocate to open doors, to enable the average person to get the best our system has to offer. I hope that one day such advocacy will not be necessary, but if it is, I hope that medical organizations such as HMOs, PPOs, insurance carriers, hospital systems and medical groups will provide their patients with advocates who can represent the interest of the patient in seeking the best we have to offer. Although this book has illustrated some of the imperfections in our healthcare system and has stressed the importance of being your own advocate or having an advocate who works on your behalf, the American healthcare system still provides exceptional care in a high-quality format usually provided by well-educated, dedicated professionals. In the coming years our healthcare system will undoubtedly change. We should not tolerate much longer a system in which millions of people are denied access to excellent healthcare. Among our great strengths has been our ability to confront problems and develop innovative solutions. I believe we will do so and provide even more exceptional care to all people. I am confident that our innovative spirit will enable all of us to get well and stay well.